First AID for t

STEP 1 2025

Your Ultimate Survival Guide: Master High-Yield Concepts and Ace the USMLE Step 1 With Questions and Answers

Grover M. Dean

Copyright © 2025 Grover M. Dean - All rights reserved.

No part of this book may be reproduced, distributed, or transmitted in any form or by any means, including photocopying, recording, or other electronic or mechanical methods, without the prior written permission of the publisher, except in the case of brief quotations embodied in critical reviews and certain other non-commercial uses permitted by copyright law.

Contents

Introduction 1

Section 1 2

Foundations of Medicine 2

    USMLE meaning 2

    History of Cell Biology 7

    Molecular Biology and Genetics 11

    What is Biochemistry? 58

    What is Immunology? 60

    Pathology 63

    Pharmacology 65

Section 2 71

Systems-Based Approach 71

    What to know about the cardiovascular system 71

    Respiratory System 76

    Gastrointestinal Tract 80

    Anatomy of the Urinary System 83

    The Endocrine System 86

    The Reproductive System 89

    Musculoskeletal System 93

    Nervous System 109

    Hematology oncology 113

    Dermatologists 115

Section 3 119

Clinical Presentations 119

    General Approach to the Patient 119

    Clinical Presentation of First Aid: USMLE | Disease Diagnosis 124

Section 4 164

High-Yield Review 164

Mastering High Yield Topics for USMLE Step 1: Elite Strategies 164

Basic Principles and Tips 168

Mnemonics and Memory Aids 172

USMLE Step 1 Sample Questions And Answers 175

Section 5 209

Test-Taking Strategies 209

How To Overcome USMLE Step 1 Exam Anxiety 209

USMLE Candidates' Guide to Time Management: Effective Strategies 212

Strategies to Help You Succeed on Step 1 of the USMLE 215

List of Abbreviations 219

Laboratory Values 220

How to Create a Study Schedule for Step 1 228

Introduction

To get a license to practice medicine in the US, you have to pass the United States Medical Licensing Examination (USMLE). It tests the skills that are needed to care for patients safely and effectively, and it sets a standard for testing medical license applicants.

The USMLE is a tough, multi-step test that checks how much medical information, clinical skills, and the ability to make decisions candidates have. Step 1 is about basic medical studies like anatomy, biochemistry, microbiology, pathology, and pharmacology. Step 2 tests clinical knowledge and skills in a number of different areas. Effective study tools are important in this high-stakes setting, and First Aid has a reputation for being one of the best ways to master the large amount of information.

One thing that makes First Aid for the USMLE stand out is that it is well-organized and breaks down complicated medical topics into forms that are easy to understand. There are short explanations, high-yield facts, pictures, mnemonics, and practice questions in this book that are formatted exactly like the test. It also promotes clinical relevance and important ideas, which helps students not only study for the test but also understand how the material is used in real-life medical practice. This guide also has everything you need to know about applying to and taking the USMLE, such as who is eligible, how to register, how much it costs, the different steps you need to take, and what you can use to prepare.

This book is known for having a lot of high-yield information in a short amount of space. It is a good way to quickly review important medical ideas and clinical information that you will need to do well on the test.

Section 1

Foundations of Medicine

USMLE meaning

The United States Medical Licensing Examination, or USMLE, is the exam needed to obtain a medical license in the United States. The USMLE was created to offer a single nationwide exam that all state medical boards could utilize to grant medical licensure to allopathic physicians. It is sponsored by two non-profit organizations, the nationwide Board of Medical Examiners (NBME) and the Federation of State Medical Boards (FSMB). (Note: Osteopathic physicians use COMLEX-USA). This guarantees that all practicing allopathic doctors, irrespective of their state of practice or prior training, have fulfilled the same evaluation requirements.

The USMLE tests doctors' patient-centered skills as well as their application of concepts, knowledge, and principles. Step 1, Step 2, and Step 3 are the three multiple-choice tests that make up the exam. These are explained in greater detail in the USMLE Steps section below.

For whom is the USMLE necessary?

The USMLE is required for all practicing physicians in the United States who work in an unsupervised context (that is, outside of postgraduate study). This is due to the fact that practicing medicine requires a license, and obtaining a medical license in the US requires passing the USMLE.

The same requirements apply to graduates who qualified domestically or abroad, guaranteeing that individuals who received their training outside of the US are evaluated using the same criteria as medical school students and graduates in the US.

Who qualifies?

You must fulfill the following prerequisites both when you apply and on test day in order to be qualified to take the USMLE exam:

Step 1 and Step 2 Clinical Knowledge

One of the following categories must apply to you:

- A medical student or graduate of an MD program approved by the Liaison Committee on Medical Education (LCME) in the United States or Canada
- A medical student or graduate of a US medical school approved by the Commission on Osteopathic College Accreditation (COCA) that grants the DO degree
- A medical student or graduate of a medical school outside of the United States and Canada who satisfies additional eligibility requirements for the Educational Commission for Foreign Medical Graduates (ECFMG) and is listed in the World Directory of Medical Schools as meeting the ECFMG eligibility requirements.

Note: Students must be "officially enrolled." You will not be eligible for the USMLE if you are dismissed or withdrawn from medical school, even if you are currently appealing.

Step 3

You must have successfully finished Steps 1 and 2 of the USMLE before submitting your application in order to be eligible for Step 3.

Additionally, you need to own one of the following:

- The MD or DO degree from a US or Canadian medical school that has received LCME or COCA accreditation.
- The World Directory of Medical Schools lists medical schools outside of the US and Canada that match the ECFMG qualifying requirements and offer the MD degree equivalent. If you qualified outside of the US and Canada, you additionally need to be ECFMG Certified.

The USMLE lasts for how long?

varying 'steps' of the USMLE have varying exam lengths; the following is the length of each step:

- Step 1 takes about eight hours.
- Step 2: Clinical Knowledge: roughly nine hours
- Step 3:
  - Day 1: roughly seven hours;
  - Day 2: roughly nine hours

The section that follows contains additional details on each USMLE phase and its structure.

Steps in the USMLE

Step 1, Step 2, and Step 3 are the three multiple-choice exams that make up the USMLE. The USMLE may also be discussed in regard to Step 2 Clinical Skills, which was formerly part of Step 2 in addition to the Clinical Knowledge component but has since been eliminated.

The following information on the exam format for each section is available on the USMLE website:

USMLE Step 1 Questions

- **Time/Length:** One-day test. Seven blocks of sixty minutes each, with breaks, for a total of almost eight hours.
- **Total Amount Of Questions:** About 280 multiple-choice questions make up the total amount of questions.
- **Assessment Area**: Your capacity to apply significant, fundamental scientific ideas to clinical situations, with an emphasis on the fundamental ideas and workings of health, illness, and treatment modalities, is the assessment area.

Clinical Knowledge Questions for USMLE Step 2

- **Time/Length**: One-day test. Eight blocks of sixty minutes each, with breaks, for a total of almost nine hours.
- **Total Amount Of Questions:** About 318 multiple-choice questions make up the total amount of questions.

- **Assessment Area**: Your capacity to apply your clinical scientific knowledge, abilities, and medical knowledge—which are crucial for patient care—with an emphasis on illness prevention and health promotion is the assessment area.

Step 3 Questions on the USMLE

Over the course of two days, Step 3 is broken up into two sections: Foundations of Independent Practice (FIP) and Advanced Clinical Medicine (ACM). With an emphasis on patient treatment in ambulatory settings, it evaluates your capacity to apply medical knowledge and comprehension of biological and clinical science.

Day 1: FIP

- **Time/Length:** One-day test. Six blocks of 60 minutes each, with breaks, for a total of almost seven hours.
- **Total Amount Of Questions:** Approximately 232 multiple-choice questions make up the total amount of questions.
- **Assessment Area**: Your understanding of fundamental medical and scientific concepts necessary for providing quality care is the assessment area.

Day 2: ACM

- **Time/Length:** One-day test. Thirteen "stimulation" blocks, each lasting no more than ten or twenty minutes, and six 45-minute blocks (for the multiple-choice questions) add up to almost nine hours, including breaks.
- **Total Amount Of Questions:** About 180 multiple-choice questions and 13 computer-based case simulations (CCS) make up the total amount of questions.
- **Assessment Area**: Your capacity to use your understanding of health and illness to manage patients is the assessment area.

Timeline for the USMLE

While there isn't a set timeframe for completing the USMLE's many stages, there are some guidelines and suggestions to take into account while determining when to finish each one.

Although Steps 1 and 2 can be done in any order, it is advised that students in medical schools with LCME accreditation complete Step 1 at the conclusion of their second year and Step 2 during their fourth year.

Only after completing Steps 1 and 2 successfully may you take Step 3 of the USMLE. Before beginning Step 3, it is advised that you have finished, or be close to finishing, at least the first year of postgraduate training in an approved US graduate medical education program.

The majority of licensing bodies stipulate that you must finish Steps 1, 2, and 3 of the USMLE within seven years of passing the first step, according to the USMLE website.

Signing up

Prometric Centers administer the computer-based USMLE Step 1, Step 2 Clinical Knowledge, and Step 3 tests. Note: Only the United States and its territories manage Step 3. On their website, you can locate the Prometric Center that is closest to you.

The registration procedure differs based on your place of study and graduation as well as the various USMLE levels. The various registration routes are as follows:

Clinical Knowledge in Steps 1 and 2:

- Applicants must apply through the NBME Licensing Examination Services if they are students or graduates of US or Canadian medical schools that have earned LCME or COCA accreditation.
- Medical school students and graduates from countries other than the US or Canada can apply through the ECFMG application website.

Step 3:

- All medical school graduates who have completed Steps 1 and 2 should apply online at the FSMB.

No matter where you studied or received your degree, the application and scheduling procedures for each component of the USMLE are the same once you have registered via the proper channel. You must do the following: Choose the time frame that works best for you to take the test.

You will receive a scheduling permit; check your inbox for it.

You can schedule your exam by going to the Prometric website.

Fees

The USMLE fees for the various exam stages are as follows:

Step 1 and Step 2 Clinical Knowledge:

For students or graduates of LCME or COCA-accredited medical schools in the US or Canada, the 2021–2022 USMLE fees are as follows:

Step 1: $645

Clinical Knowledge in Step Two $645

Extension of the Eligibility Period $70

If you need to know about rescheduling fees for USMLE Steps 1, 2, and 3, go to the USMLE rescheduling fees page.

The following are the USMLE fees for medical school students and graduates who are not from the US or Canada:

Application for ECFMG	$150
Step 1	$975 + $180 international test delivery surcharge, if testing outside of the US or Canada
Step 2 Clinical Knowledge	$975 + $200 international test delivery surcharge, if testing outside of the US or Canada
Eligibility Period Extension	$90
Step 1 / Step 2 Testing Region Change	$85 per region change

Step Three

The application fee for USMLE Step 3 is non-refundable and cannot be transferred between applications or eligibility periods.

The cost for 2021 is $895.

For additional details regarding international fees, please consult the USMLE website.

Supplies you'll need

To aid with your exam preparation, the USMLE website offers a variety of "practice materials," such as

- general information booklets and content descriptions.
- Sample questions and supplies for tests
- Practice test items and tutors

To assist you become used to the test center setting, they also provide the option of taking a practice exam at a Prometric test center; however, this service comes with a cost.

Practice problems for the USMLE

Using practice questions and mock exams in addition to the practice materials and sample questions on the USMLE website will help you get a feel for the kinds of questions you'll encounter on the test and give you the chance to hone your answering abilities.

Soon to come...

Our USMLE questions are customized for you and concentrate on your areas for improvement using cutting-edge algorithms that automatically determine your strengths and limitations. enabling you to advance more quickly and utilize your USMLE preparation time more efficiently.

Following USMLE

You will be eligible to apply for a license to practice medicine after passing Step 1, Step 2, Clinical Knowledge, and Step 3 of the USMLE. You can practice in an unsupervised environment (i.e., outside of postgraduate training) thanks to this.

History of Cell Biology

The basic building block of life is a single cell, which can exist alone (unicellular organisms) or join to generate multicellular organisms, according to contemporary cell biology. However, how did we get to this realization? Let's start with a brief overview of cell biology.

An Overview of Cell Structure in Brief

Let's quickly review the fundamental structure of individual cells before delving into the history of cell biology.

There are many different kinds of cells, ranging from eukaryotic plant and animal cells to prokaryotic ones like bacteria and archaea. Red blood cells, neurons, and epithelial cells are just a few of the more unique cell types that fall under these categories.

Depending on their cell specialization, these different cell types have different structures. Nonetheless, one characteristic that distinguishes cells is their membranes. These are necessary to keep the cell's environment constant. They control the flow of substances into and out of the cell across the membrane.

DNA, or deoxyribonucleic acid, is the genetic substance found in the majority of cells. DNA is kept in a subcellular space called the nucleus in eukaryotes.

DNA is found in the cytoplasm of prokaryotes, which lack intracellular membranes. Mature red blood cells are among the cell types with particular functions that do not include DNA. The general anatomy of both prokaryotic and eukaryotic cells is depicted in Figure 1.

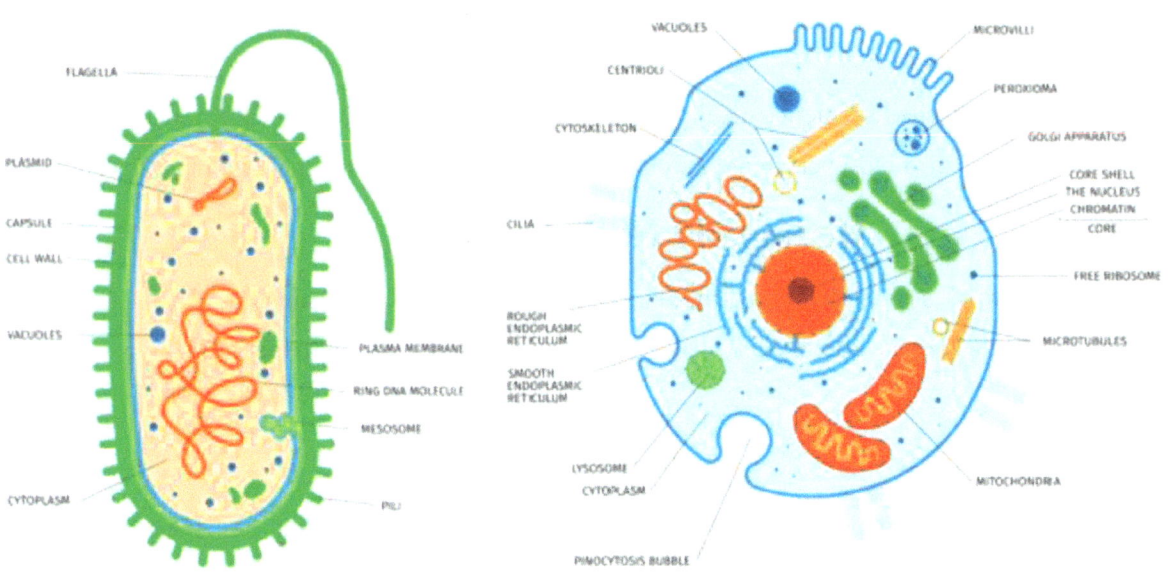

Figure 1. comparison between prokaryotic and eukaryotic cells' general structures.

The Cell Theory

All organisms are made up of similar basic units of organization called cells, according to the cell hypothesis, often known as the cell doctrine. The idea has remained the cornerstone of contemporary biology since Schleiden & Schwann formally introduced it in 1839. Other major biological paradigms, such as Darwin's theory of evolution (1859), Mendel's laws of heredity (1865), and the development of comparative biochemistry (1940), were all preceded by this concept.

The First Cells in Cork

The development of the telescope allowed humans to observe the cosmos, but the light microscope revealed the composition of living forms and allowed for the exploration of smaller worlds. Robert Hooke made the initial discovery of the cell and gave it its name in 1665. The name came from his observation that it resembled the tiny chambers known as cellula, which were occupied by monks.

But what Robert Hooke truly observed under a microscope were the dead cell walls of plant cells, or cork. When Hooke described these cells, Micrographia published his work. Hooke's observations of cell walls did not reveal the nucleus and other organelles present in the majority of living cells.

When he described the algae Spirogyra in 1674, Anton van Leeuwenhoek became the first person to see a live cell under a microscope. Van Leeuwenhoek most likely observed microbes as well.

Development of the Cell Theory

Theodor Schwann and Matthias Jakob Schleiden were discussing their cell research while sipping coffee after supper in 1838. Schwann may have been impressed by the resemblance between plant cells and animal cells he had seen in tissues when he heard Matthias Schleiden describe plant cells with nuclei.

Without delay, the two scientists proceeded to Schwann's lab to examine his slides. The following year saw the publication of Schwann's book on animal and plant cells (Schwann 1839), which did not acknowledge Schleiden's or anyone else's contributions (1838). He distilled his findings concerning cells into three conclusions:

1. The basic unit of organization, physiology, and structure of living organisms is the cell.
2. The cell continues to exist as both an independent entity and a component of living things.
3. Similar to how crystals develop (spontaneous generation), cells form by free-cell creation.

The third principle is obviously incorrect, but the first two are still true as of right now. Rudolph Virchow's influential maxim, Omnis cellula e cellula, which states that "all cells only arise from pre-existing cells," eventually supported the proper understanding of cell formation by division and was formally stated in that statement.

Contemporary Theory of Cells

1. Cells make up all known living things.
2. The cell is the structural & functional unit of all living things.
3. All cells come from pre-existing cells by division. (Spontaneous Generation does not occur).
4. Hereditary information is stored in cells and is transferred from one cell to another during cell division.
5. In terms of their chemical makeup, all cells are essentially identical.
6. Cells are the site of all life's energy flow, including metabolism and biochemistry.

The 1950s saw an explosion in cell biology research, similar to the explosive expansion of molecular biology in the middle of the 20th century. Maintaining, growing, and modifying cells outside of living things became feasible.

Using cervical cancer cells from Henrietta Lacks, who passed away from her disease in 1951, George Otto Gey and associates created the first continuous cell line to be thus cultivated in 1951. The cell line, later known as HeLa cells, has been a turning point in the study of cell biology, much like the structure of DNA was a major discovery in molecular biology.

Amidst a wave of advancements in cell research, the next ten years saw the development of sterile cell culture methods and the characterization of the minimal medium requirements for cells. The discovery of green fluorescent protein in jellyfish, the development of transfection techniques, the discovery of short interfering RNA (siRNA), and earlier developments in electron microscopy all contributed to its success.

Today, cytology, a field of biology, is dedicated to the study of cell structure and function. Particularly in the clinical setting, this subject has advanced thanks to equipment advancements like cytology microscopes and reagents.

The Chronology of Cell Biology History

A chronology of some significant occasions in the evolution of cell theory and cell biology may be seen below.

Jansen is credited with creating the first compound microscope in 1595.

In 1655, Hooke wrote about "cells" in cork.

Protozoa were discovered by Leeuwenhoek in 1674. Nine years or so later, he discovered bacteria.

Brown described the cell nucleus in orchid cells in 1833.

Cell theory was put forth by Schleiden and Schwann in 1838.

Albrecht von Roelliker discovered that egg and sperm cells are also cells in 1840.

1856. N. Pringsheim saw how an egg cell was pierced by a sperm cell.

In 1858, anthropologist, pathologist, and physician Rudolf Virchow explains his well-known finding: omnis cellula e cellula, which states that cells only develop from preexisting cells.

Kolliker first spoke of mitochondria in 1857.

Flemming explained how chromosomes behave during mitosis in 1879.

1883: The chromosomal theory of heredity states that germ cells are haploid.

Golgi described the Golgi apparatus in 1898.

1938: To separate cytoplasm from nuclei, Behrens employed differential centrifugation...

The first commercial transmission electron microscope was made by Siemens in 1939.

Gey and associates created a continuous human cell line in 1952.

The dietary requirements of animal cells in culture were methodically established by Eagle in 1955.

In order to separate nucleic acids, Meselson, Stahl, and Vinograd invented density gradient centrifugation in cesium chloride solutions in 1957.

In 1965, Ham unveiled a specific serum-free medium. The first scanning electron microscope sold commercially was made by Cambridge Instruments.

1976: Research by Sato and associates demonstrates that various cell lines need distinct hormone and growth factor combinations in serum-free medium.

1981 saw the creation of fruit flies and transgenic mice. An embryonic stem cell line was created in mice.

1995: A GFP mutant with improved spectral characteristics is discovered by Tsien.

1998 saw the cloning of mice from somatic cells.

SiRNA was identified by Hamilton and Baulcombe in 1999 as a component of post-transcriptional gene silencing (PTGS) in plants.

2006: The necessary elements for the production of induced pluripotent stem cells are found, enabling the differentiation of differentiated cells into stem cells.

2009: Single-cell sequencing is introduced, providing information on transcriptomics at the cell level.

2009 saw the publication of the first study to use organoids made from a single adult stem cell.

2012: The development of CRISPR gene editing enables precise genome engineering that targets RNA.

A Synopsis of Cell Biology History

Numerous distinct scientific and technological advancements have occurred throughout the history of cell biology, ranging from the development of the microscope, which allowed us to view individual cells, to the identification of fluorescent proteins and the creation of potent electron microscopes, which allowed us to conduct more in-depth research on the structure and function of cells.

With the advent of microscopes, the majority of people can now observe cells up close.

Molecular Biology and Genetics

Molecular and Cellular

The Life Molecules

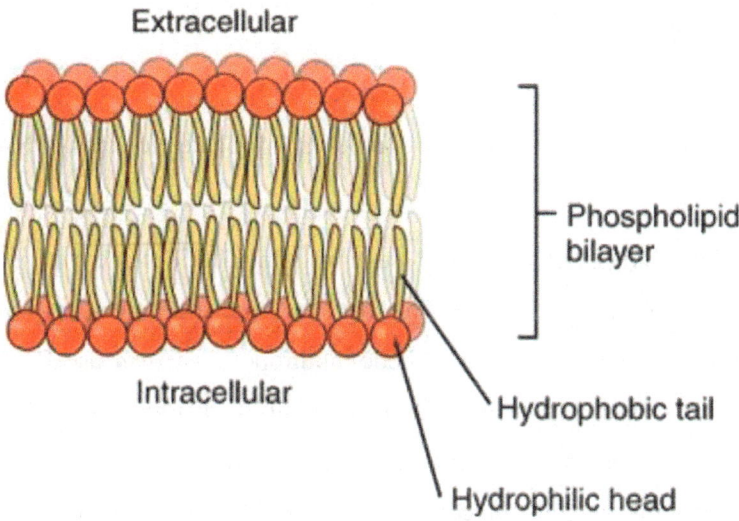

Figure 3.1 shows phospholipid molecules with hydrophilic heads and hydrophobic tails forming a bilayer.

The four fundamental chemical types that make up organisms—proteins, lipids, carbohydrates, and nucleic acids—are necessary for the construction and operation of cells. Often folded into intricate three-dimensional shapes, proteins are made up of chains of amino acids. A hydrophilic (loving water) head and a hydrophobic (repelling water) tail characterize the structure of lipids (Figure 3.1). Lipids combine to generate fats and triglycerides, which are more complicated molecules. An organism can obtain energy by breaking down the carbon and hydrogen atoms that make up carbohydrates. Finally, the genetic information of a living thing is carried by nucleic acids.

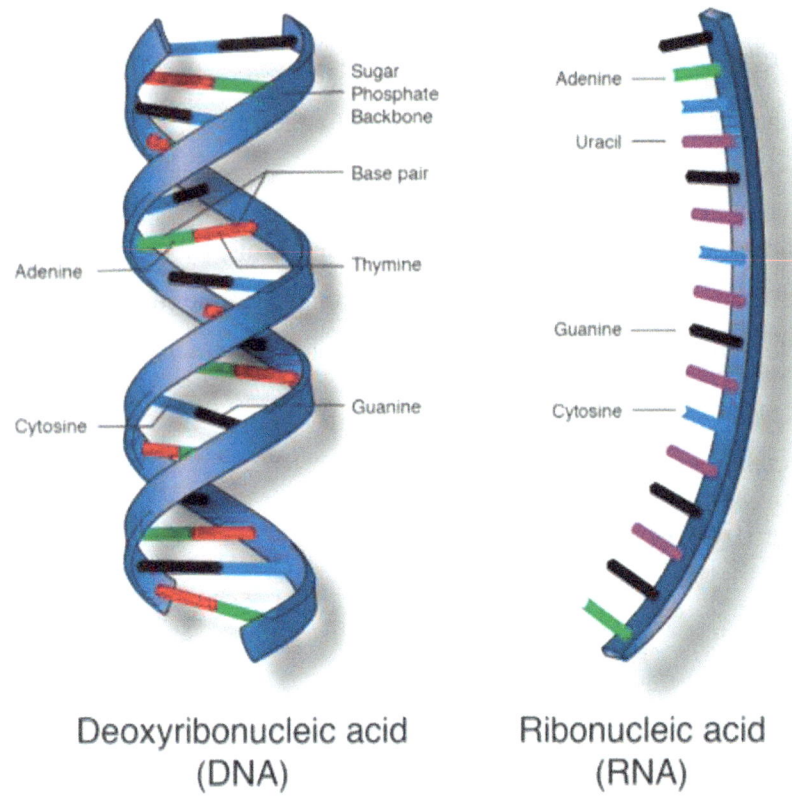

Figure 3.2: The structural elements that combine to make either single-stranded or double-stranded nucleic acids (DNA and RNA).

Probably the most familiar nucleic acid is deoxyribonucleic acid (DNA). DNA is made up of nucleotides and a sugar-phosphate backbone (Figure 3.2). The physical structure of DNA and the information that DNA nucleotides give will be covered in more detail later.) Because each organism has its own DNA genetic code, anthropologists can use DNA nucleotide sequences to identify the relationships between various organisms. By examining 20 distinct short DNA sequences known as "CODIS Core Loci," forensic investigators can identify individuals in the case of humans. Ribonucleic acid (RNA) is another type of nucleic acid. Proteins are constructed by chaining amino acids together using a particular kind of RNA molecule (Figure 3.3 and Figure 3.4). Later in the chapter, we'll go over how RNA turns amino acids into proteins.

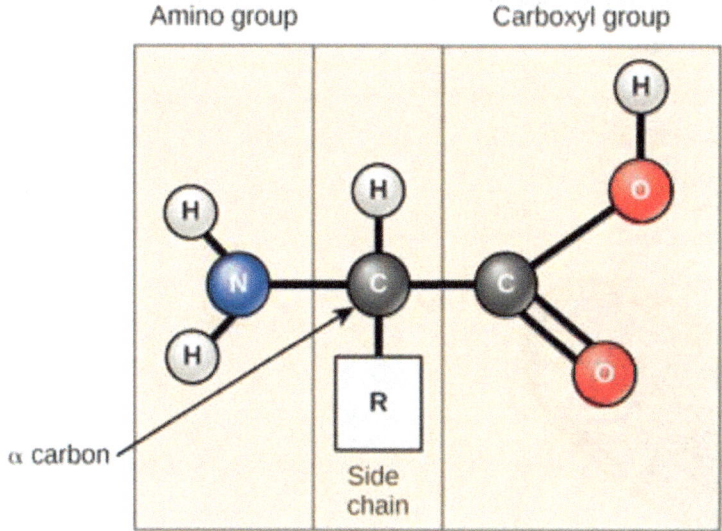

Figure 3.3 lists the chemical components that define an amino acid. N: nitrogen; O: oxygen; H: hydrogen; C: carbon.

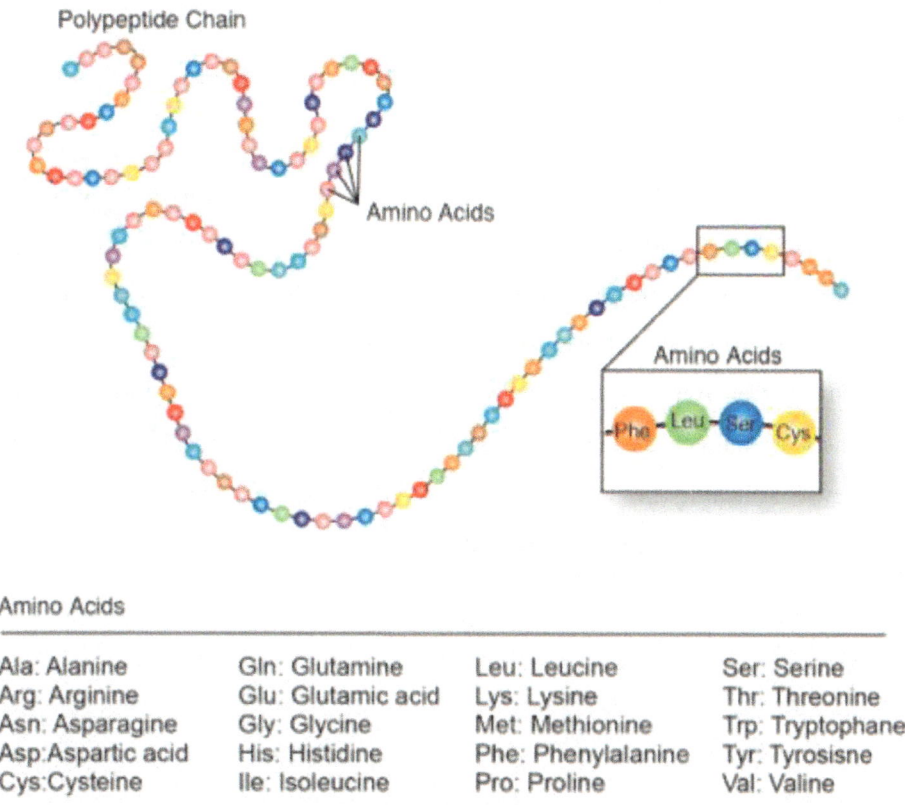

Figure 3.4 Amino acids (20 different types) strung together form a polypeptide chain.

The cells

Using a microscope, Robert Hooke examined slices of plant cork in 1665. According to Hooke, the minute plant structures he observed looked like cella, which is Latin for "a small room." Approximately two centuries later, biologists

13

recognized the cell as being the most fundamental unit of life and that all life is formed of cells. Cellular organisms can be described as two basic cell types: prokaryotes and eukaryotes.

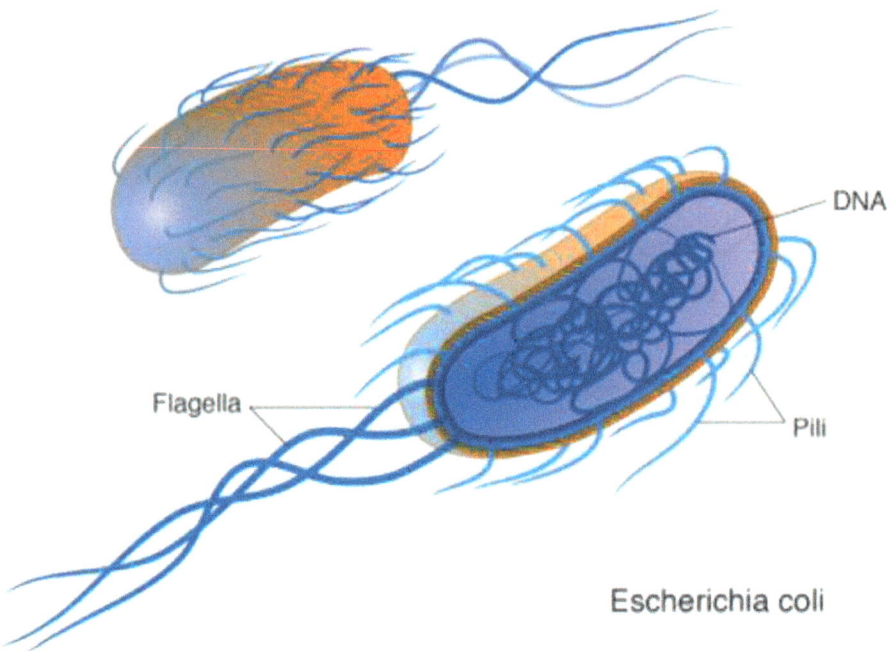

Figure 3.5: An illustration of E's single-celled body. coli bacterium.

Prokaryotes, which are made up of a single cell, include bacteria and archaea. They also lack separate membranes around their organelles and DNA. As a result, their DNA and the remainder of the cell are not separated by any compartments (Figure 3.5). The fact that certain bacteria can make people sick is well recognized. Salmonella and Escherichia coli (E. coli) infection, for example, can cause symptoms of food poisoning. Strep throat and pneumonia are brought on by streptococcal germs. One bacterial sexually transmitted illness is Neisseria gonorrhoeae. Even though bacteria are frequently linked to disease, not all of them are dangerous. For instance, the connection between human health and the microbiota is being investigated by experts. A healthy human microbiome includes bacteria that aid in food digestion, strengthen the immune system, and even produce vitamins (such B12 and K).

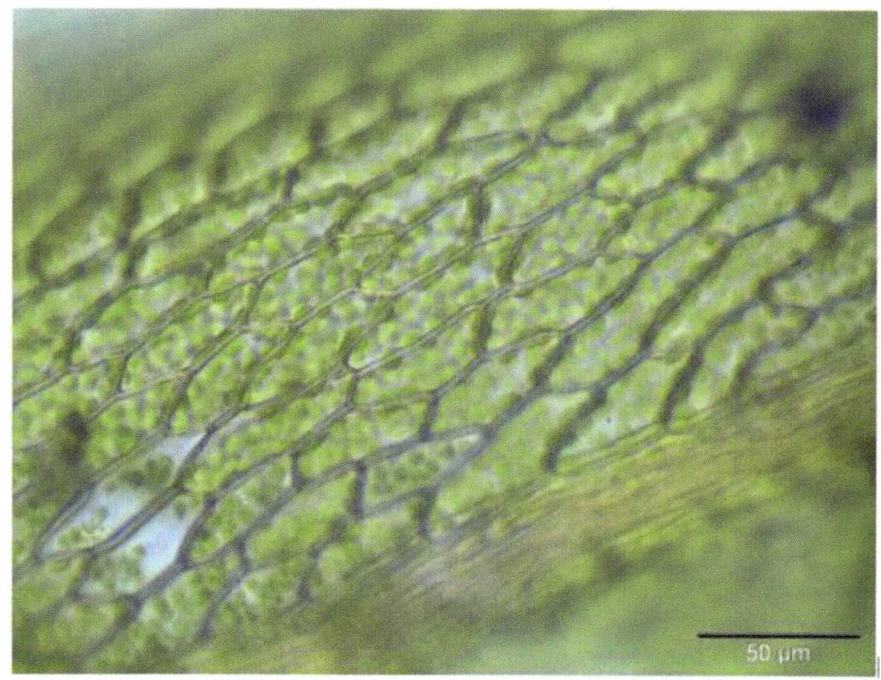

Figure 3.6 shows the membranes of plant cells under a microscope.

Bacteria and the second class of prokaryotic organisms, the archaea, were once thought to be closely linked. But once genomic investigation revealed that archaea have a unique evolutionary ancestry, biologists categorized them into a different taxonomic realm. Because they were found to live in harsh conditions, archaea are referred to as "extremophiles." For instance, archaea can be found in hot climates, like Yellowstone National Park's Old Faithful Geyser.

Single-celled or multicelled organisms are examples of eukaryotes. Eukaryotes have membranes enclosing their organelles and DNA, unlike prokaryotes. Microscopic algae called phytoplankton, which can create oxygen from the sun, are an example of a single-celled eukaryote. Fungi can be single- or multicellular, and yeasts are also single-celled. Both plants and animals have many cells.

Despite the startling parallels between plant and animal cells, there are also some significant variances. For instance, the thick outer cell wall of plant cells is composed of cellulose, a fibrous carbohydrate (Figure 3.6). The tissues of plant and animal cells differ as well. A collection of similar-looking cells that carry out the same function is called a tissue. The outermost layer of cells in most plants generates a waxy cuticle that protects the cells and stops them from losing water. However, humans have skin, the outermost cell layer of which is largely composed of a tough protein called keratin. Overall, humans have a multitude of tissue types (e.g., cartilage, brain, and heart).

Organelles of Animal Cells

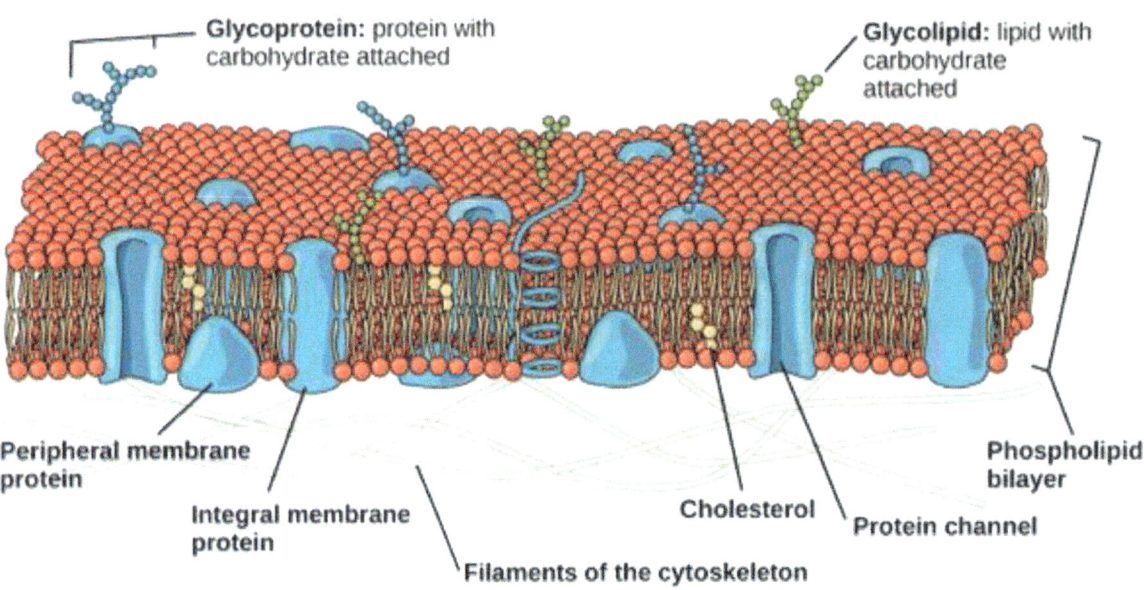

Figure 3.7 A phospholipid bilayer with membrane-bound carbohydrates and proteins.

A double membrane known as the phospholipid bilayer envelops an animal cell (Figure 3.7). The lipids and proteins that make up this protective barrier provide cellular processes structure and function, as a closer examination demonstrates. For example, lipids and proteins embedded in the cell's membrane work together to govern the movement of molecules and ions (e.g., H2O and sodium) into and out of the cell. Cytoplasm is the jelly-like matrix inside of the cell membrane. Organelles are a component of the cytoplasm and serve the cell in a variety of specific capacities (Figure 3.8). The cell's DNA is found in the nucleus, which is an example of an organelle (Figure 3.9). The nuclear envelope, the double membrane that surrounds the nucleus, acts as a barrier to preserve the integrity of DNA and controls the flow of chemicals into and out of the nucleus.

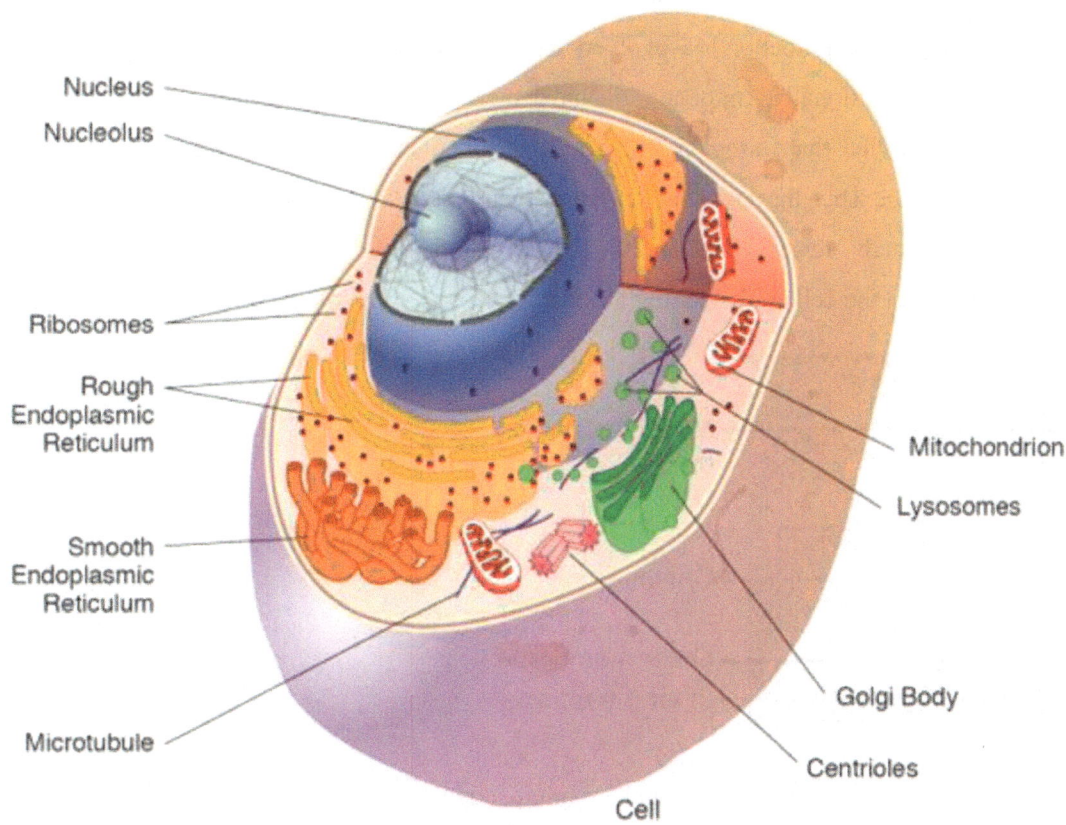

Figure 3.8: An animal cell with organelles contained by membranes.

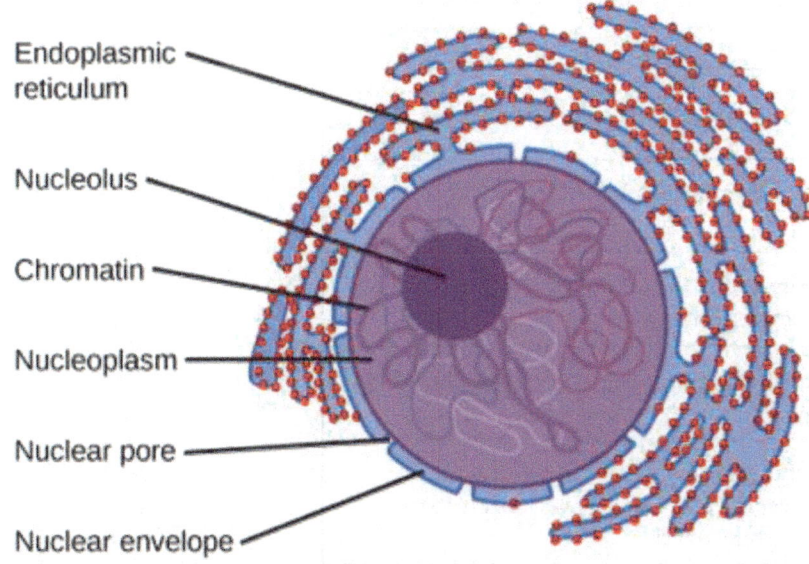

Figure 3.9 An animal cell's nucleus enclosed by a membrane.

Figure 3.10 shows the mitochondrion, another crucial organelle. The reason mitochondria are frequently called "powerhouse centers" is because they generate adenosine triphosphate (ATP), which is the cell's energy source. The number of mitochondria in each cell of multicellular eukaryotes can range from hundreds to thousands, depending on the species and tissue type. Researchers have concluded that the development of the eukaryotic cell was significantly influenced by mitochondria. Over time, mitochondria evolved into cellular organelles from symbiotic prokaryotic organisms, or beneficial bacteria. Additionally, mitochondria have their own DNA, known as mitochondrial DNA (mtDNA), which is explained by the fact that mitochondria were once distinct species. All organelles have crucial physiological roles, and illness may arise when they are unable to carry them out as well they can. Cells with mitochondrial disorders, for instance, contain abnormally fewer mitochondria. This results in a variety of neurological symptoms and illnesses in people. Other organelles in the cell are listed together with their specific biological functions in Figure 3.11.

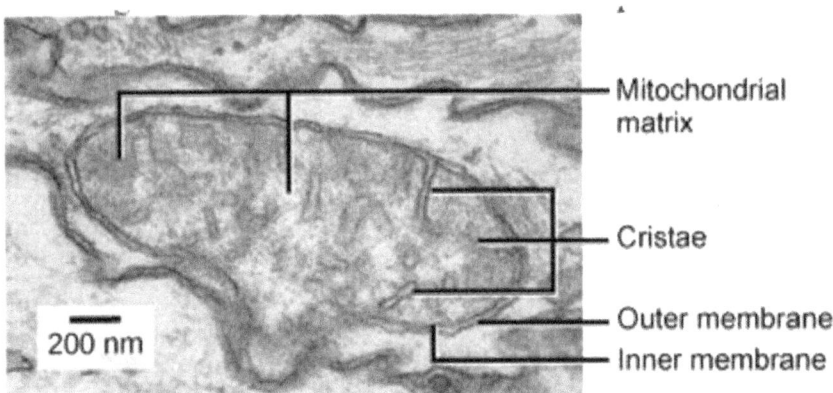

Figure 3.10 An mammalian mitochondrion organelle seen under a microscope.

Cell structure	Description
Cytoplasm	Fluid substance located inside of cell membrane that contains organelles
Nucleopore	Pores in the nuclear envelope that are selectively permeable
Nucleus	Contains the cell's DNA and is surrounded by the nuclear envelope
Nucleolus	Resides inside of the nucleus and is the site of ribosomal RNA (rRNA) transcription, processing, and assembly
Mitochondrion	Responsible for cellular respiration, where energy is produced by converting nutrients into ATP
Ribosome	Located in the cytoplasm and also the membrane of the rough endoplasmic reticulum. Messenger RNA (mRNA) binds to ribosomes and proteins are synthesized
Endoplasmic reticulum (ER)	Continuous membrane with the nucleus that helps transport, synthesize, modify, and fold proteins. Rough ER has embedded ribosomes, whereas smooth ER lacks ribosomes

Golgi body	Layers of flattened sacs that receive and transmit messages from the ER to secrete and transport proteins within the cell
Lysosome	Located in the cytoplasm and contains enzymes to degrade cellular components
Microtubule	Involved with cellular movement including intracellular transport and cell division
Centrioles	Assist with the organization of mitotic spindles which extend and contract for the purpose of cellular movement during mitosis and meiosis

Figure 3.11 lists the names of the organelles together with their biological roles.

GENETICS INTRODUCTION

The study of heredity is called genetics. Offspring inherit the genetic characteristics of their parents. Even while children look like their parents, their characteristics can differ in terms of appearance or molecular function. Red-green colorblindness, for instance, can occasionally be produced in a son by two parents with normal color vision. A later part will address genetic inheritance patterns. Molecular geneticists investigate the biological processes—such as DNA mutations (see Chapter 4), cell division, and genetic regulation—that produce individual variety.

To test anthropological hypotheses, molecular anthropologists employ genetic data. Molecular anthropology research encompasses a wide range of topics, but some of them include human origins, dispersals, evolution, adaptation, demography, health, disease, behavior, and animal domestication. Molecular anthropologists not only study in labs but also interact with various communities of people in the field. Additionally, some anthropologists examine the DNA of people who have been dead for decades, or even hundreds or thousands of years. Through the study of ancient DNA (aDNA), certain laboratory methods have been developed. Thorough methodological considerations must be made because the DNA in ancient people's skeletons deteriorates (becomes less intact) over time. Chapter 10 will provide an example of an aDNA study, whereas Special Topic: Native American Immunity and European Diseases offers a current example.

Special Topic: An Examination of Ancient DNA in Relation to Native American Immunity and European Illnesses

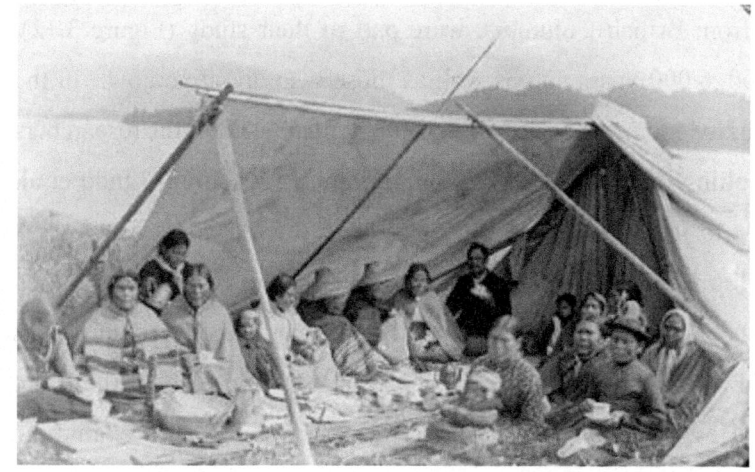

Pacific Northwest Coast Tsimshian Native Americans (Figure 3.12a).

Due to foreign nations' colonization, Native Americans gradually experienced significant death rates starting in the early 15th century. The main cause of the decline in the number of indigenous peoples in the Americas is European-borne illnesses like smallpox, influenza, TB, and measles. In addition to living in densely populated, sedentary communities, many European immigrants to the New World had also had to deal with pests and domestic animals. Despite the fact that some prehistoric Native American cultures (particularly in Mesoamerica) may be classified as big agricultural societies, their subsistence methods, communal living, and general culture differed significantly from those of Europeans. Native Americans are therefore thought to have been vulnerable to old-world diseases because they did not live in the same urban settings as Europeans.

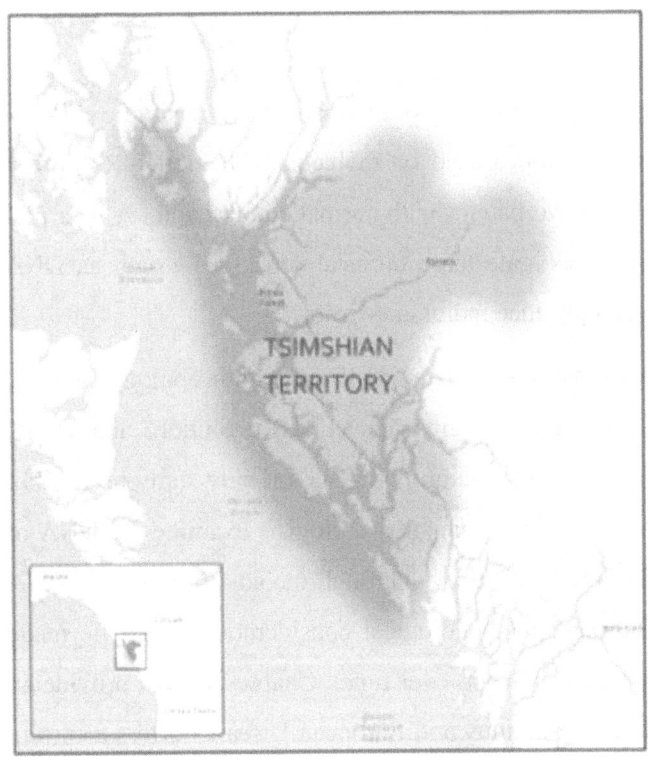

British Columbia's Tsimshian area (Figure 3.12b).

Whether pre-contact Native Americans had a genetic predisposition to European diseases was first examined in a 2016 Nature publication. Tsimshians, a First Nation group from British Columbia, were part of their study (Figure 3.12). Analysis was done on the DNA of people who lived 500–6,000 years ago as well as those who are alive now. In the genetic region HLADQ-1, one of the major histocompatibility complex (MHC) immune system molecules, the researchers found a mutation. These molecules are in charge of spotting infections and starting an immune reaction. Lindo et al. (2016) found that Native Americans were able to adjust to their local natural ecology with the aid of HLADQ-1. A particular HLADQ-1 DNA pattern linked to ancient Tsimshian immunity, however, was no longer adaptive when European-borne diseases struck the Northwest in the 1800s. The frequency of HLADQ-1 sequences in modern Tsimshians is different due to previous selection pressures from European diseases. We still need to learn more about the exact function of HLADQ-1 in immunological adaptability. However, taken as a whole, this study shows how examining ancient DNA from the remains of people who have passed away can shed light on historical events and current human populations.

DNA Contains Genetic Information

It is surprising to learn that the study of inheritance came before the discovery of DNA. It was once thought that the genetic information passed down from parents to children was contained in proteins. The effectiveness of their bacterial genetic research was then linked to isolated nucleic acids by Oswald Avery, Colin MacLeod, and Maclyn McCarty in 1944. They specifically showed that their pneumonia bacterial strains' genetic change was caused by the molecule DNA. Their discoveries were not entirely accepted by the field of molecular biology, despite the fact that their study was groundbreaking at the time (it has also been speculated that they were ignored for a Nobel Prize). The scientific world soon came to agree that DNA is an organism's genetic material, particularly after the molecular structure of DNA was discovered.

The structure of DNA

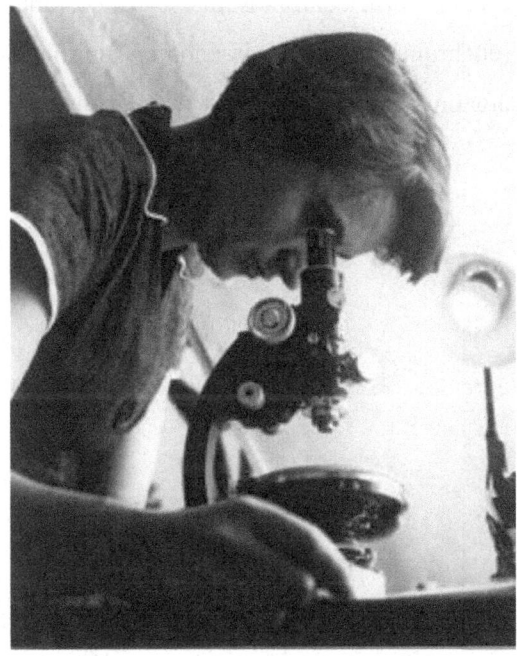

Figure 3.13 Rosalind Franklin, a chemist and X-ray crystallographer.

The 1953 discovery of the molecular structure of DNA was one of the greatest scientific breakthroughs of all time. Using X-ray crystallography, Rosalind Franklin (Figure 3.13) generated the image that clearly indicated the double helix form of DNA. But because the revelation caused so much debate, Franklin's colleague and outside associates got more attention. Maurice Wilkins, Francis Crick, and James Watson were awarded the Nobel Prize in 1962 for creating a biochemical model of DNA. Unfortunately, ovarian cancer claimed Rosalind Franklin's life in 1958. Franklin is now generally recognized for her significant contribution and her standing as a highly accomplished scientist.

One way to think of DNA's double helix form is as a twisted ladder (see Figure 3.2). The two strands of DNA are oriented in opposite directions, or antiparallel, making it a double-stranded molecule. Each strand has a sugar-phosphate backbone and is made up of nucleotides. DNA nucleotides come in four varieties: adenine (A), thymine (T), cytosine (C), and guanine (G). Chemical bonding rules between nucleotide base pairs hold the two DNA strands together. According to the complementary base-pairing rules, C and G form a bond, whereas A and T bond with one another. Because of the "weak" interactions between the hydrogen atoms that form the chemical bonds between A—T and C—G, the two strands are easily separated. A DNA sequence is the arrangement of the nucleotide bases (A, T, G, and C) on a single strand of DNA. One DNA strand will have the complementary sequence GTACGA if the other strand has the sequence CATGCT. An illustration of a brief DNA sequence is this. Human cells actually contain over three billion DNA base pairs.

The nucleus contains highly organized DNA.

It would be roughly two meters (6.5 feet) long if the DNA from a single human cell were taken out and stretched out entirely. DNA molecules must thus be arranged in the nucleus in a compact manner. The double helix structure of DNA coils to do this. An example would be to twist a string until coils form, then twist it again to create secondary coils, and so on. DNA first wraps itself around proteins known as histones to help coil. As a result, chromatin—which looks like "beads on a string"—is formed (Figure 3.14). The chromatin then coils even more to form a chromosome. Chromosomes can change from being tightly coiled (chromatin) to being loosely coiled (euchromatin), which is another significant characteristic of DNA. Chromosomes in the nucleus often stay in a euchromatin state, which makes DNA sequences available for regulatory activities.

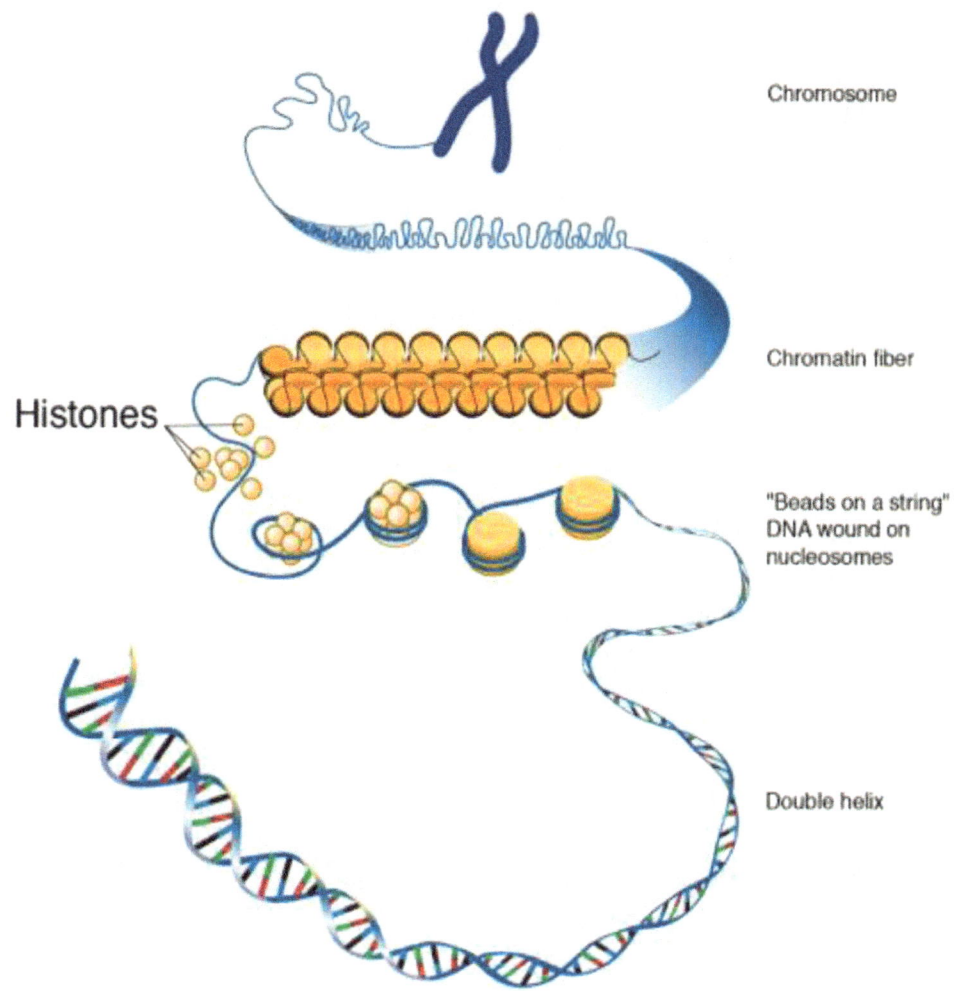

3.14 The hierarchical arrangement of chromosomes.

In the nucleus of each human body cell, there are 46 chromosomes, which are typically arranged in 23 pairs (Figure 3.15). An intriguing fact is that the quantity of chromosomes an organism possesses is not contingent upon the complexity or magnitude of the organism. For example, hermit crabs possess 254 chromosomes, whereas chimpanzees possess 48. In addition, centromeres (the "centers") and telomeres (the extremities) are distinct physical structures of chromosomes (Figure 3.16). Chromosomes are defined as having two distinct "arms," one of which is longer and the other shorter, as a result of centromeres. The subsequent section will address the significance of centromeres in the process of cell division. Telomeres are situated at the termini of chromosomes and are responsible for safeguarding the chromosomes from degradation following each round of cell division. Nevertheless, as we age, our telomeres become shorter, and if the chromosome telomeres become excessively short, the cell will cease to divide. Consequently, researchers are highly intrigued by the correlation between the regulation of telomere length and cellular senescence.

Chromosomes of the Human Genome

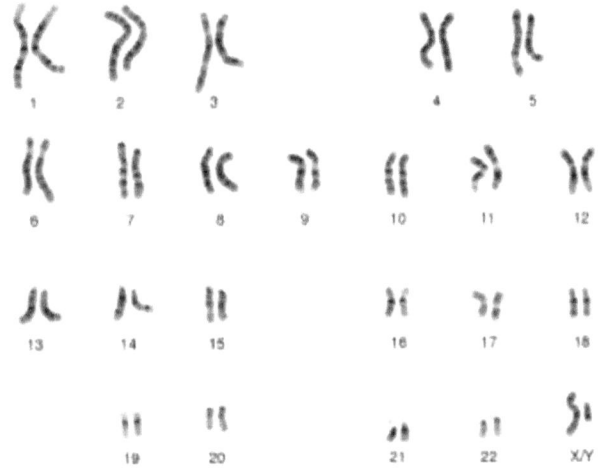

Figure 3.15 illustrates the 23 pairs of human chromosomes.

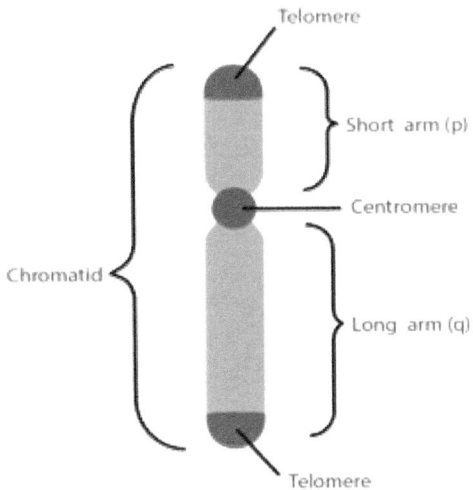

Figure 3.16 illustrates the regions of a chromosome.

DNA REPLICATION AND CELL DIVISION

In order for life to persist and thrive, cells must be capable of dividing. It is also essential for the preservation of an organism throughout its lifespan to promote tissue growth and the repair of cellular injury. All of these are contingent upon the dynamic processes of DNA replication and the cell cycle. The mechanisms that are emphasized in this section are highly regulated and only comprise a portion of a cell's life cycle.

DNA Replication

DNA replication is the process by which new DNA is copied from an original DNA template. It is a phase of the highly coordinated cell cycle that necessitates a diverse array of enzymes with unique functions. Enzymes are responsible for the high-energy and structural reactions that are involved in the replication of a double helical molecule. Semi-conservative replication is the term used to characterize the process of generating a complementary DNA strand from a template strand. The outcome of semi-conservative replication is the formation of two distinct double-stranded DNA structures, each of which is comprised of a newly synthesized "daughter" DNA strand and an original "parent" template strand.

Initiation, elongation, and termination are the three stages through which DNA replication proceeds. DNA replication commences with the recruitment of enzymes to specific locations along the DNA sequence, which is referred to as initiation. For instance, the double helix of DNA poses structural obstacles to replication. Consequently, an initiator enzyme known as helicase "unwinds" DNA by disrupting the hydrogen bonds between the two progenitor strands. The active site of the replication apparatus is the fork, which is formed by the unraveling of the helix into two separated strands (Figure 3.17). The progenitor template strands are exposed, allowing for their reading and replication, once both strands have been separated.

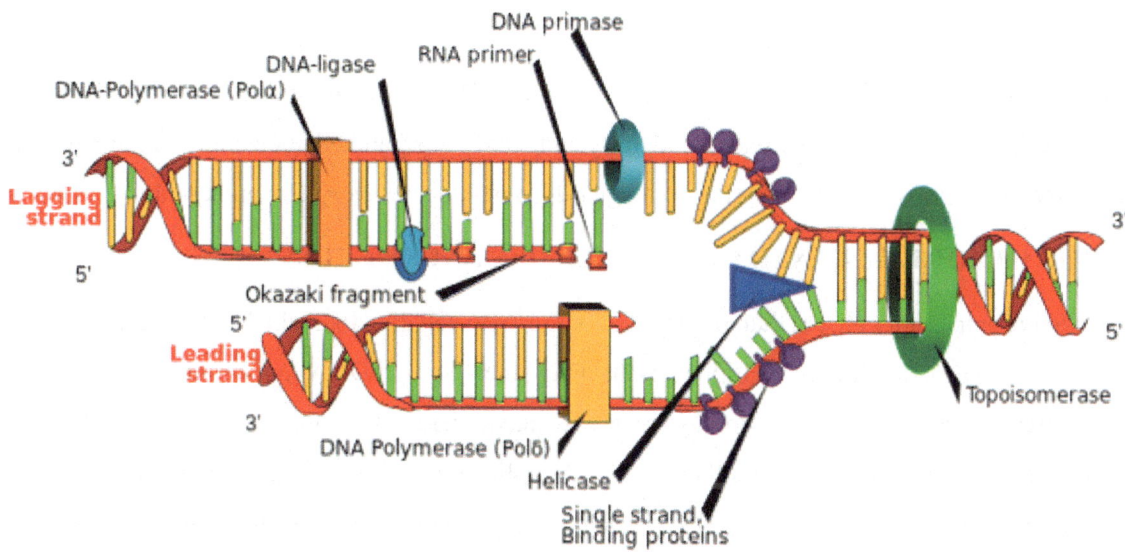

Figure 3.17 illustrates the various enzymes that are linked to DNA replication.

Elongation defines the process of forming new DNA offspring strands from parent strands. The two progenitor strands can be further classified as either the leading strand or the lagging strand, as indicated by the direction of replication, which is either continuous or discontinuous. A primer is a brief fragment of RNA nucleotides that attaches to the parent DNA strand that will be copied. One primer is administered to the leading strand, while the lagging strand is administered multiple primers. DNA polymerases, which read parent template strands in a specific direction, assist in the process of elongation. The newly formed daughter strand will grow as complementary nucleotides are introduced. The direction of replication is contingent upon whether it is the leading or lagging strand. A single continuous strand will be generated by a DNA polymerase on the leading progenitor strand. Disjointed strands, known as Okazaki fragments, will be produced due to the fact that the lagging parent strand necessitates multiple primers. The nucleotide openings between the disconnected lagging strand Okazaki fragments will be filled in by other enzymes.

Lastly, termination denotes the conclusion of DNA replication activity. This is indicated by a stop sequence in the DNA, which is identified by the apparatus at the replication fork. The final outcome of DNA replication is that the number of chromosomes is doubled, allowing the cell to divide into two.

DNA Mutations

The replication of DNA should lead to the formation of two molecules that possess identical DNA nucleotide sequences. Copying errors are estimated to occur every 10^7 DNA nucleotides, despite the fact that DNA polymerases are highly precise during DNA replication. A mutation is a deviation from the original DNA sequence. Chapter 4 will provide a more comprehensive examination of the various forms of mutations. In summary, mutations can lead to the insertion or deletion of nucleotides and repeated sequences, as well as single nucleotide alterations. Mutations may be deleterious (hazardous) depending on their location. For instance, cancer may arise as a consequence of mutations in regions that regulate the cell cycle (see Special Topic: The Cell Cycle and Immortality of Cancer Cells). Nevertheless, numerous additional mutations are not detrimental to an organism.

The cell endeavors to decrease the frequency of mutations that occur during DNA replication, irrespective of their impact. Polymerases with proofreading capabilities are available to identify and rectify mismatched nucleotides in order to achieve this. The frequency of DNA mutations is reduced by these safeguards to only occur every 10^9 nucleotides.

SPECIAL TOPIC: THE IMMORTALITY AND CELL CYCLE OF CANCER CELLS

DNA replication is one of the preparatory phases that a cell undergoes prior to cell division, which are collectively referred to as interphase (Figure 3.18). The cell not only multiplies its chromosomes through DNA replication during interphase, but it also enhances its metabolic capacity to supply energy for growth and division. Proteins that function as checkpoints strictly regulate the transition into each phase of the cell cycle. DNA replication and/or cell division will not proceed if a cell is unable to overcome a checkpoint. DNA damage, insufficient size, or a lack of nutrients to continue the process are among the reasons a cell may fail at a checkpoint. Subsequently, apoptosis, a mechanism for cell demise, may be implemented by a cell.

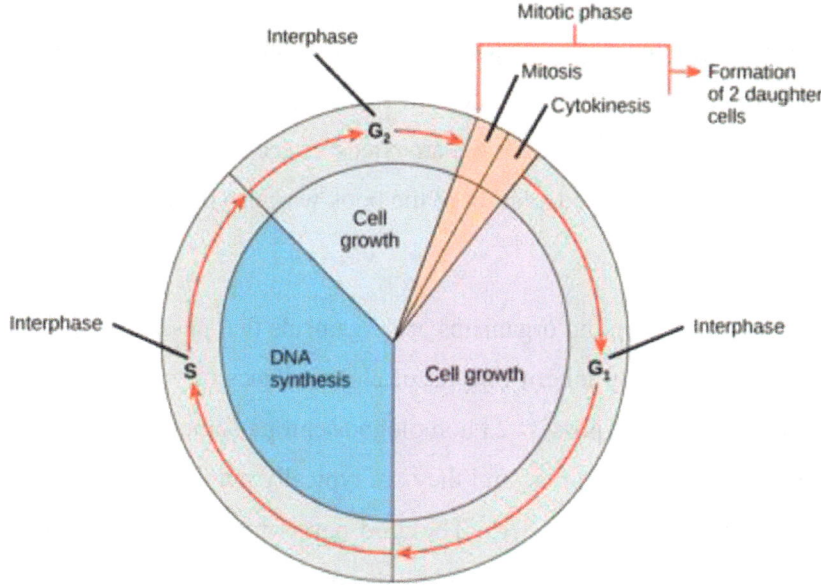

The phases and milestones of the cell cycle are illustrated in Figure 3.18.

Cancer is characterized by unbridled cellular proliferation. In other words, cancer cells develop the ability to evade death and replicate indefinitely as they grow and proliferate. This uncontrolled and continuous cell division is also referred to as "immortality." As previously mentioned, the majority of cells lose the capacity to divide as a result of the telomeres' shortening at the extremities of chromosomes over time. The length of their telomeres is perpetually protected, which is one method by which cancer cells maintain replicative immortality. Chemotherapy is frequently employed to combat cancer by inhibiting the proliferation of genetically abnormal cells through the targeting of cell division. Another therapeutic approach that is currently under investigation is the targeting of telomere activity to halt the division of cancer cells.

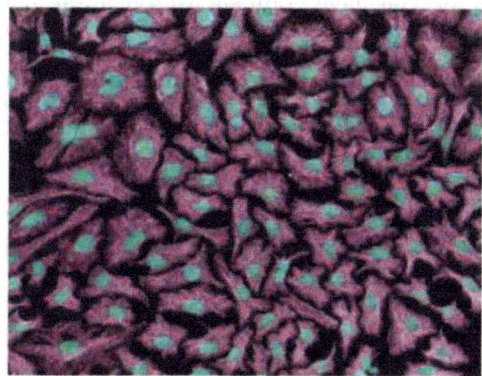

A microscopic slide of HeLa carcinoma cells is depicted in Figure 3.19.

The immortality of cancer cells has been leveraged by researchers to conduct molecular research. HeLa cells (Figure 3.19) are the earliest immortal cell line. They were obtained from Henrietta Lacks, an African-American woman who was diagnosed with cervical cancer in 1955. HeLa cells continued to replicate, despite the fact that extracted cells frequently perished during experiments at that time. The propagation of Lacks's cell line has made a substantial contribution to medical research, including the ongoing study of cancer and the testing of the polio vaccine in the 1950s. Regrettably, Lacks had not provided her consent for the use of her tumor biopsy in cell culture research. Additionally, her family was unaware of the remarkable application and extraction of her cells for two decades. In 1976, the early history of HeLa cell origin was disclosed. In 2010, The Immortal Life of Henrietta Lacks, published an extensive account of HeLa cells that included the controversy raised by the Lacks family. In 2017, a film adaptation of the book was also published.

Mitotic Cell Division

Somatic cells constitute the organism and its diverse tissues. Diploid organisms are organisms that possess two sets of chromosomes in their somatic cells. Humans are diploid, as they inherit one set of chromosomes (n = 23) from each parent, resulting in a total of 46 chromosomes. Consequently, they possess 23 homologous chromosomes, which are also referred to as matching pairs. The size of these homologous pairs varies, and they are typically numbered from largest (chromosome 1) to smallest (chromosome 22), as illustrated in Figure 3.15. The 23rd pair, which consists of the sex chromosomes (X and Y), is an exception. The female sex is typically represented by the symbol XX, while the male sex is represented by the symbol XY. An X chromosome is inherited from the mother, while an X or Y chromosome is inherited from the father.

Somatic cells must divide in order to develop and repair tissues. In order for cell division to take place, a cell must first replicate its genetic material, as previously mentioned. Each chromosome generates twice the quantity of genetic information during DNA replication. Sister chromatids are the duplicated limbs of chromosomes that are attached at the centromeric region. To clarify, the number of chromosomes remains constant at 46; however, the cell's genetic material is doubled as a consequence of replication.

Mitosis is the process of somatic cell division that results in the formation of two diploid progeny cells. Mitosis is briefly illustrated in Figure 3.20. Mitotic spindle fibers (microtubules) facilitate chromosomal movement by adhering to the centromeric region of each chromosome after DNA and other constituents in the cell have completed replication. In particular, the spindle fibers physically align each chromosome at the cell's center. Subsequently, the spindle fibers separate the sister chromatids and relocate each to the opposite side of the cell. During this phase, the cell contains 46 chromosomes on each side. The cell is now capable of dividing into two daughter cells that are fully separated.

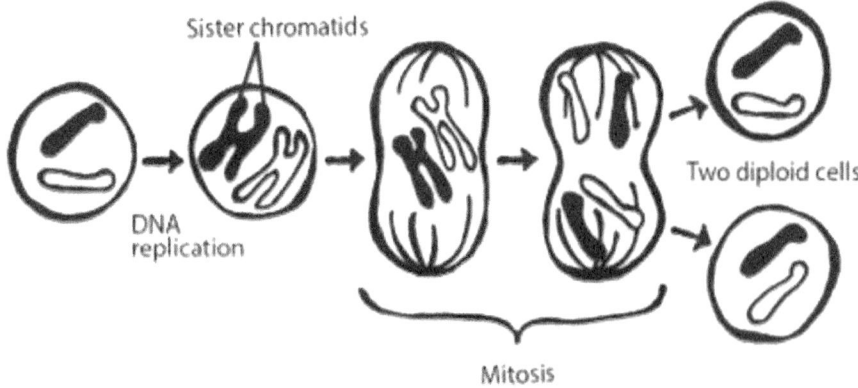

Figure 3.20 illustrates the process of mitotic cell division.

Meiotic Cell Division

Gametogenesis is the process of producing gametes, which are composed of sperm and egg cells. This process entails two cycles of cell division, known as meiosis. The progenitor cell in meiosis is diploid, similar to mitosis. Nevertheless, meiosis exhibits a few significant distinctions, such as the quantity of daughter cells produced (four cells, which necessitate two cycles of cell division to generate) and the number of chromosomes each daughter cell possesses (Figure 3.21). Each chromosome ($n = 46$) replicates its DNA during the initial round of division, which is referred to as meiosis I. This process results in the formation of sister chromatids. Subsequently, spindle fibers facilitate the alignment of homologous chromosomes in the vicinity of the cell's center, thereby enabling sister chromatids to exchange genetic material. In other words, the sister chromatids of chromosomes that are identical cross over at the same DNA nucleotide position. Genetic recombination is the process by which homologous chromosomes cross over, exchange DNA, and subsequently rejoin segments. The "genetic shuffling" that takes place in gametes enhances the genetic diversity of organisms by generating novel combinations of genes on chromosomes that are distinct from those of the progenitor cell. Recombination can also result in the formation of genetic mutations. For instance, the two sister chromatids may undergo an unequal exchange of genetic material, which may lead to the deletion or duplication of DNA nucleotides. After the completion of genetic recombination, homologous chromosomes are separated, resulting in the formation of two daughter cells.

The progeny cells that remain after the initial round of meiosis are haploid, which is to say that they possess only one set of chromosomes ($n = 23$). Sister chromatids are separated and two additional haploid daughter cells are formed during the second round of cell division, which is referred to as meiosis II. Consequently, the four daughter cells that result have a genetic composition that is not identical to that of the parent cells or to each other, as well as a single set of chromosomes ($n = 23$).

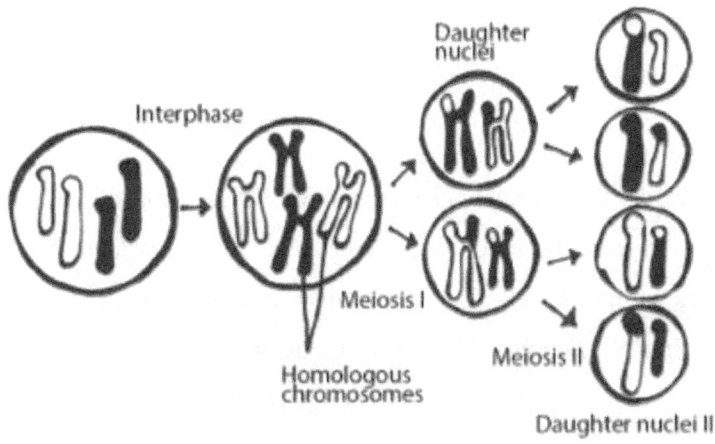

Figure 3.21 illustrates the division of meiotic cells.

Despite the fact that both sperm and egg gamete production undergo meiosis, the ultimate number of viable daughter cells varies. Four mature sperm cells are generated during spermatogenesis. Although four egg cells are also generated during oogenesis, only one of these egg cells will produce a mature egg, or ovum. During fertilization, a diploid cell is formed by the fusion of an egg cell and sperm cell, which subsequently develops into an embryo. The ovum also contains the cellular organelles that are essential for the division of embryonic cells. This encompasses mitochondria, which is the reason why humans and the majority of other multicellular eukaryotes possess the identical mtDNA sequence as their mothers.

Disorders of the Chromosome

Errors may result in the complete deletion or duplication of chromosomes during mitosis or meiosis. For instance, homologous chromosomes may not separate properly, resulting in one daughter cell possessing an excess chromosome and the other daughter cell possessing an extra chromosome. Aneuploid cells are characterized by an abnormal or unexpected number of chromosomes. Karyotyping is a method that can be used to determine the number of chromosomes in adult or embryonic cells. Aneuploid cells are generally detrimental to the division of a cell or the development of an embryo, which can result in the loss of pregnancy. Nevertheless, Down Syndrome, a genetic condition characterized by the presence of three copies of the 21st chromosome, is relatively prevalent. Additionally, human males and females may be born with aneuploid sex chromosome conditions, including XXY, XXX, and XO, which all refer to a single X chromosome.

PROTEIN SYNTHESIS

Proteins were initially defined as strings of amino acids that fold into intricate 3-dimensional structures at the outset of the chapter. In humans, there are 20 standard amino acids that can be arranged in a variety of ways, allowing proteins to perform a remarkable number of distinct functions. For example, muscle fibers are proteins that aid in the facilitation of movement. Immunoglobulins, a distinct category of proteins, assist in the protection of the organism by identifying disease-causing pathogens within the body. Physiological activity is regulated by protein hormones, including insulin. A protein known as blood hemoglobin is responsible for the transportation of oxygen throughout the body. Enzymes are proteins that serve as mediators for biochemical reactions within the cell, including metabolism. Protein structures that are larger in scale can be observed as tangible characteristics of an organism, such as hair and nails.

Transcription and Translation

The specifications for the production of proteins are provided by the coding nucleotides in our DNA. Transcription and translation are the two primary stages in the process of protein synthesis, which is also known as protein production. The synthesis of protein is contingent upon numerous molecules within the cell, such as various types of regulatory proteins and RNAs, for each stage of the process. Messenger RNA (mRNA) will be the primary focus of our discussion, despite the fact that there are numerous types of RNA molecules that serve a diverse array of functions within the cell.

A gene is a DNA segment that encodes RNA, and its length can range from a few hundred to as many as two million base pairs. The objective of transcription is to generate an RNA copy of the genetic code (Figure 3.22). RNA molecules are single-stranded nucleotide sequences, in contrast to double-stranded DNA (refer to Figure 3.2). Furthermore, DNA is composed of the nucleotide thymine (T), whereas RNA lacks it. RNA's fourth nucleotide is uracil (U). Uracil is complementary to adenine (A) or can form a pair with it, whereas cytosine (C) and guanine (G) remain complementary to one another. In order for transcription to occur, the cell must first activate a gene (see Special Topic: Genetic Regulation of the Lactase (LCT) Gene for a more comprehensive discussion of gene regulation). The double-stranded DNA is subsequently separated, and one side of the DNA strand is employed as a template for the assembly of complementary RNA nucleotides. For instance, the newly generated mRNA sequence will be AUGCCUACG if the DNA template is TACGGATGC. The transcribed RNA is occasionally the final product required by the cell; however, the initial step in protein synthesis is the construction of pre-messenger RNA (pre-mRNA).

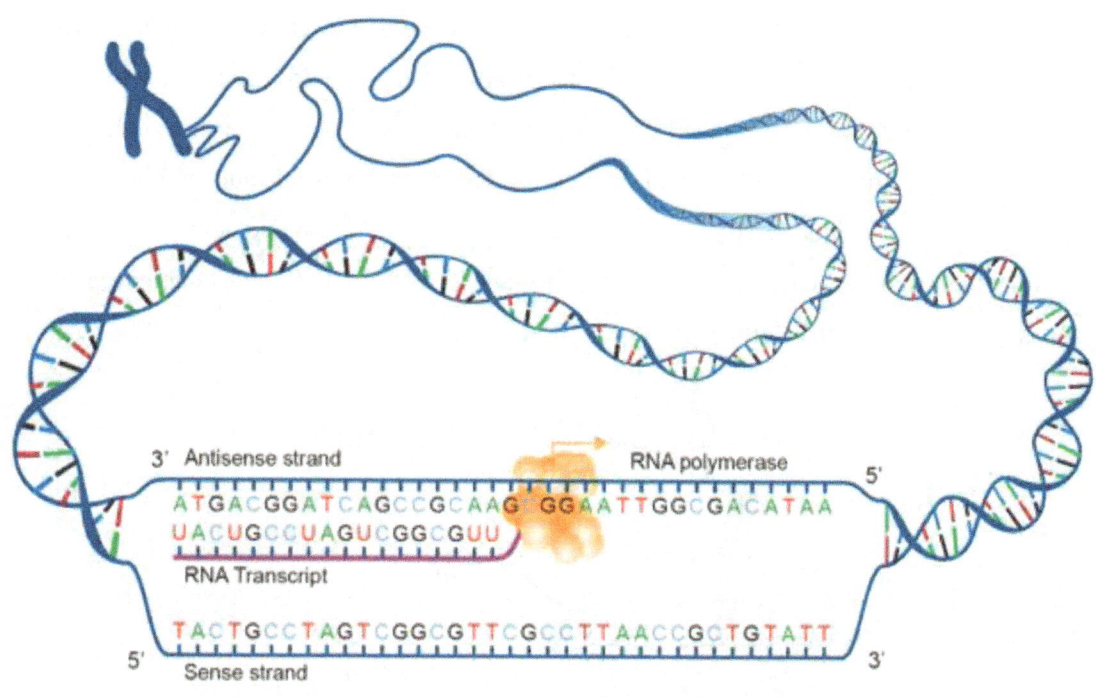

Figure 3.22 illustrates the process of DNA transcription catalyzed by RNA polymerase.

Introns and exons are segments that are present in genes. Exons are classified as "coding" and introns as "noncoding," which implies that the information they contain is not required for the production of proteins. Introns and exons are both present during the initial transcription of a gene into pre-mRNA (Figure 3.23). Nevertheless, introns are eliminated through a process known as splicing after transcription is completed. A protein/RNA complex attaches to the pre-mRNA during splicing, removing introns and connecting the remaining exons to form a truncated mature mRNA.

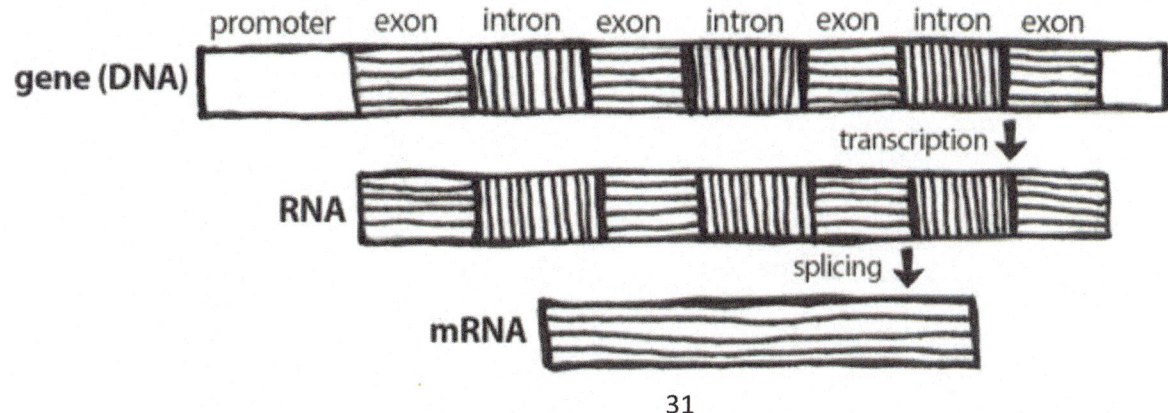

Figure 3.23 illustrates the process of RNA processing, which involves the removal of introns, a process known as splicing, between transcription and translation.

Translation is the process by which amino acids are chained together to create new proteins after mRNA is "read." Mature mRNA is transported outside of the nucleus during translation, where it is bound to a ribosome (Figure 3.24). The nucleotides in the mRNA are read as triplets, which are referred to as codons. The premise for the construction of a protein is the correspondence between each codon and an amino acid. In accordance with the preceding example, the mRNA sequence AUG-CCU-ACG encodes three amino acids. AUG is a codon for methionine (Met), CCU is a codon for proline (Pro), and ACG is a codon for threonine (Thr) when a codon table is employed (Figure 3.25). Consequently, the protein sequence is Met-Pro-Thr. Methionine is the most frequently encountered "start codon" (AUG) for the commencement of protein translation in eukaryotes. The amino acid chain that is expanding departs the ribosome and folds into a protein as the ribosome advances along the mRNA (Figure 3.26). The ribosome ceases to add new amino acids, detaches from the mRNA, and the protein is released when it reaches a "stop" codon (UAA, UAG, or UGA). Proteins that have been folded can be employed to accomplish a structural or functional function.

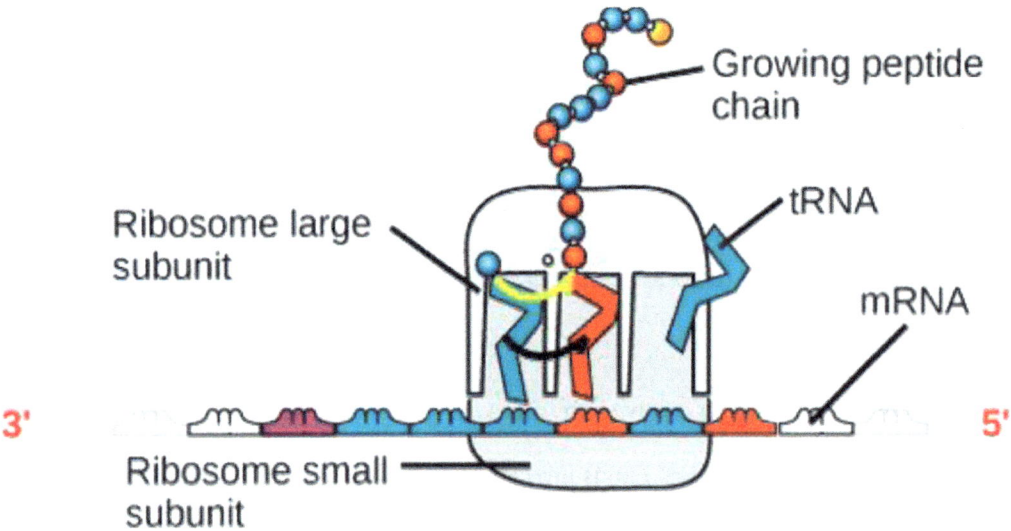

Figure 3.24 illustrates the translation of mRNA into an amino acid.

RNA codon table

1st position	2nd position U	2nd position C	2nd position A	2nd position G	3rd position
U	Phe	Ser	Tyr	Cys	U
U	Phe	Ser	Tyr	Cys	C
U	Leu	Ser	stop	stop	A
U	Leu	Ser	stop	Trp	G
C	Leu	Pro	His	Arg	U
C	Leu	Pro	His	Arg	C
C	Leu	Pro	Gln	Arg	A
C	Leu	Pro	Gln	Arg	G
A	Ile	Thr	Asn	Ser	U
A	Ile	Thr	Asn	Ser	C
A	Ile	Thr	Lys	Arg	A
A	Met	Thr	Lys	Arg	G
G	Val	Ala	Asp	Gly	U
G	Val	Ala	Asp	Gly	C
G	Val	Ala	Glu	Gly	A
G	Val	Ala	Glu	Gly	G

Amino Acids

Ala: Alanine
Arg: Arginine
Asn: Asparagine
Asp: Aspartic acid
Cys: Cysteine
Gln: Glutamine
Glu: Glutamic acid
Gly: Glycine
His: Histidine
Ile: Isoleucine
Leu: Leucine
Lys: Lysine
Met: Methionine
Phe: Phenylalanine
Pro: Proline
Ser: Serine
Thr: Threonine
Trp: Tryptophane
Tyr: Tyrosisne
Val: Valine

Figure 3.25 This table can be employed to determine the mRNA codons (sequence of three nucleotides) that correspond to each of the 20 distinct amino acids. For instance, if the codon is CAU, the first position is "C" and you would examine the corresponding row. The second position is "A" and you would examine the corresponding column. The third position, "U," narrows the row and signifies that the CAU codon corresponds to the amino acid "histidine" (abbreviated "His"). The table also displays the three "stop" codons (UAA, UAG, or UGA) and the most prevalent "start codon" (AUG) that is associated with Methionine.

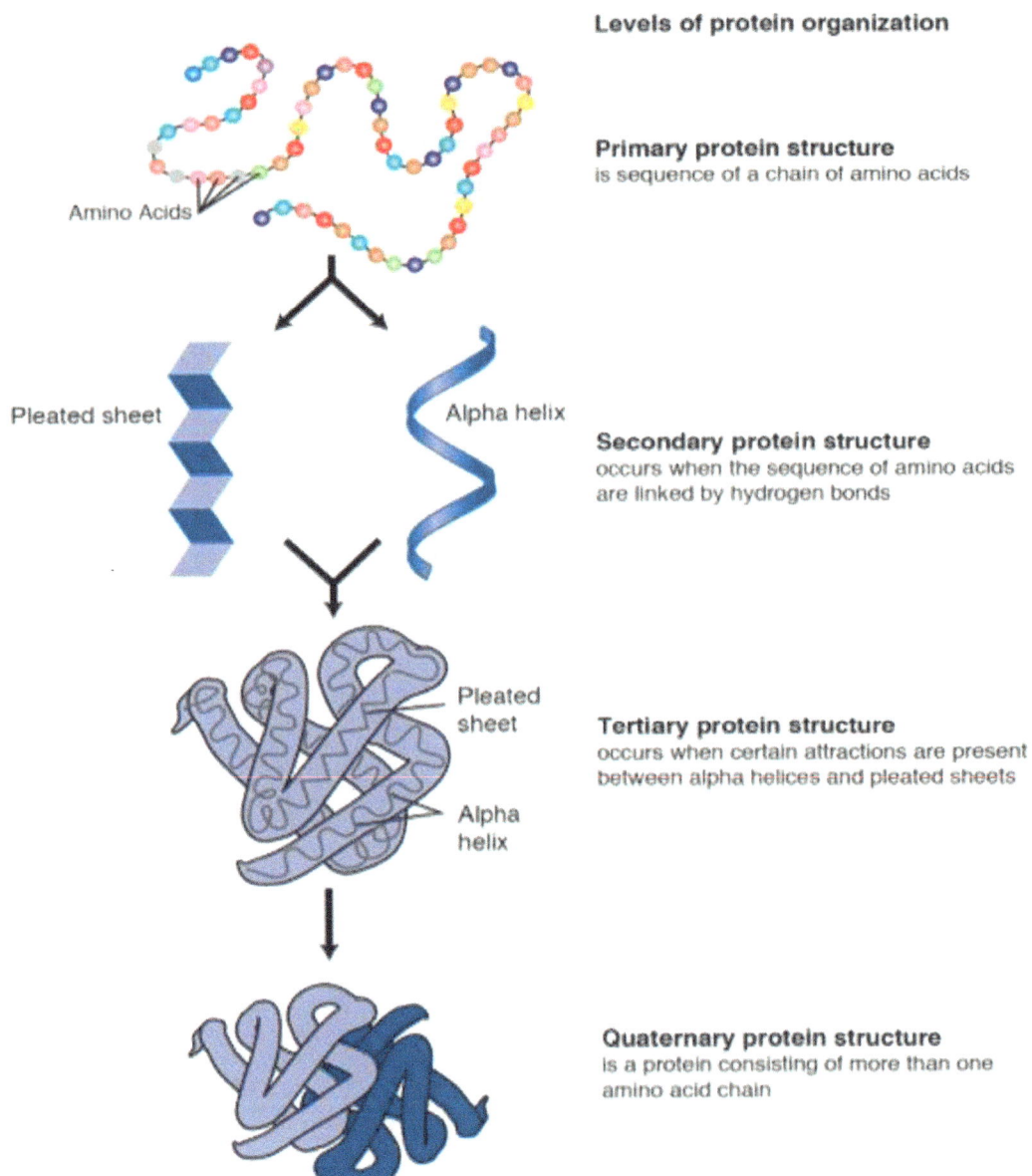

The protein organization is depicted in Figure 3.26, beginning with the simple amino acid chain, which is subsequently pleated and organized into more complex protein structures.

SPECIAL TOPIC: THE GENETIC REGULATION OF THE LACTASE (LCT) GENE

The lactase protein, which is synthesized in the small intestine, is encoded by the LCT gene. It is accountable for the degradation of lactose, a substance that is present in milk. Lactose intolerance is characterized by an insufficient production of lactase enzyme, which results in the development of digestive symptoms. Individuals may avoid milk products wholly, consume lactose-free milk, or take lactase supplements to prevent this discomfort.

An effective illustration of the mechanism by which cells regulate protein synthesis is the LCT gene. Whether or not the LCT gene is transcribed is regulated by the promoter region, which is either "on" or "off." The production of lactase is triggered by the binding of a regulatory protein, a transcription factor, to a specific site on the LCT promoter. The RNA polymerases are subsequently recruited, and they read DNA to link together nucleotides to produce RNA molecules (Figure 3.22). In the nucleus, an LCT pre-mRNA is synthesized, and additional chemical modifications are applied to the extremities of the mRNA to prevent its degradation within the cell.

The subsequent step is the processing of RNA. The mature mRNA is produced by a spliceosome complex that connects exons and removes introns. The LCT mRNA is bound to a ribosome, a multi-protein complex that includes ribosomal RNA (rRNA), after it is transported outside of the nucleus. The ribosome of eukaryotes is composed of two primary subunits: the smaller bottom subunit, which has a binding site for mRNA, and the larger top subunit, which contains transfer RNA (tRNA) binding sites (see Figure 3.24). A nucleotide anticodon is present in each tRNA and is capable of recognizing an mRNA codon. Upon binding to an mRNA codon in the ribosome, a tRNA transfers the corresponding amino acid. The correct order of linking the newly introduced amino acid is guaranteed by rRNA. The lactase enzyme, which is capable of decomposing lactose, is subsequently formed by the folding of the developing protein.

The decrease in transcriptional "silence" of the LCT gene over time is the primary cause of the loss of milk digestion in the majority of animals as they mature. Nevertheless, certain individuals possess the capacity to metabolize lactose into adulthood, a condition referred to as "lactase persistence." This implies that they possess a genetic mutation that results in the continuous transcription of LCT. Lactase persistence mutations are prevalent in populations that have a long history of pastoral husbandry, such as those in northern Europe and North Africa. It is hypothesized that lactase persistence developed as a result of the nutritional advantages of milk digestion.

Mendelian genetics and other inheritance patterns

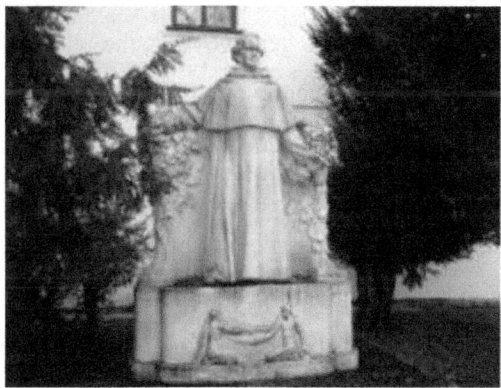

Figure 3.27 depicts the Mendel statue, which is situated at the Mendel Museum at Masaryk.

Gregor Johann Mendel (1822–1884) is frequently referred to as the "Father of Genetics." Mendel, a priest, conducted pea plant breeding experiments in a monastery situated in the present-day Czech Republic (Figure 3.27). Mendel presented his research to a local scientific community in 1865 and published his findings the following year, following several years of experimentation. Despite the fact that his meticulous effort was noteworthy, the significance of his work was not acknowledged for an additional 35 years. One of the reasons for the delay in recognition is that his findings did not align with the prevailing scientific perspectives on inheritance at the time. For instance, it was once believed that the physical characteristics of parents were "combined" and that their offspring inherited an intermediate form of the trait. Conversely, Mendel demonstrated that specific physical characteristics of pea plants (such as flower color) were individually transmitted to the subsequent generation in a statistically predictable manner. Mendel also noted that certain parental traits disappeared in progeny but subsequently reemerged in subsequent generations. He elucidated this phenomenon by introducing the concepts of "dominant" and "recessive" attributes. The following section provides a review of some of the fundamental laws of inheritance that Mendel established. Additionally, Mendelian genetics is the term used to describe the examination of traits and diseases that are regulated by a single gene.

Mendelian Genetics

Seed		Flower	Pod		Stem	
Form	Cotyledons	Color	Form	Color	Place	Size
ROUND	YELLOW	WHITE	FULL	YELLOW	AXIAL FLOWERS	TALL
WRINKLED	GREEN	PURPLE	CONSTRICTED	GREEN	TERMINAL FLOWERS	SHORT

Figure 3.28: Different genotypes of pea plants produce a range of phenotypic traits.

A trait's physical manifestation is referred to as an organism's phenotype. Mendel examined the phenotypes of the pea plant (Pisum sativum), which are depicted in Figure 3.28. In each of these instances, a single gene governs the physical characteristics. According to Mendelian genetics, an organism's genotype determines its phenotype. Two gene copies make up a genotype, with one copy coming from each parent. Since they are located in the same gene locus on homologous chromosomes, gene copies are also referred to as alleles (Figure 3.29). Because of their various DNA sequences, alleles can have varying phenotypic effects. In other words, depending on which two alleles (i.e., genotypes) an organism carries, multiple phenotypes may be produced even though alleles code for the same feature. Mendel's pea plants, for instance, all contain blooms, yet they can be either purple or white. Therefore, the two color alleles that are present in a genotype determine the color of the flower.

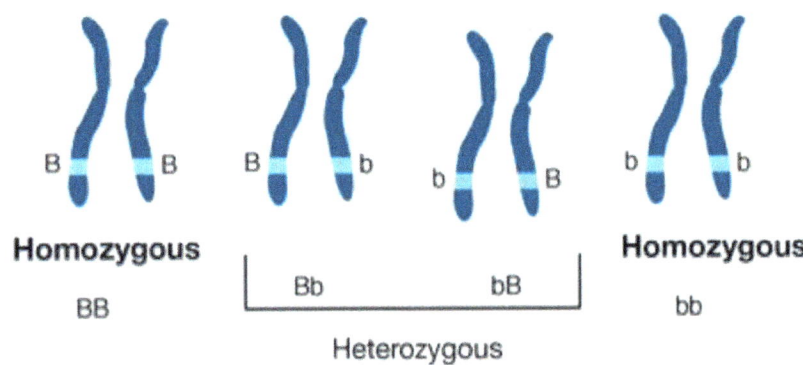

36

The various homozygous and heterozygous combinations that can result from two distinct alleles (B and b) are depicted in Figure 3.29, which shows homologous chromosome pairings.

One graphic that can be used to illustrate Mendelian inheritance patterns is the Punnett square. A Punnett square, for example, can be used to forecast the ratio of Mendelian genotypes and phenotypes that an offspring of parents with known genotypes would have. A Punnett square with two heterozygous parents for blossom color (Bb) is shown in Figure 3.30. Two distinct alleles for the same gene are known as a heterozygous genotype. As a result, a pea plant with one purple allele and one white allele is heterozygous for flower color. Two copies of the same allele make up an organism's genotype when it is homozygous for a certain trait. The two heterozygous parents of the pea plants can have heterozygous (Bb) or two distinct homozygous genotypes (BB or bb) in their progeny, as shown in the Punnett square example (Figure 3.30).

The potential genetic combinations of children from two heterozygous parents are shown in Figure 3.30, a Punnett square.

A purple-flowered pea plant may be homozygous (BB) or heterozygous (Bb). This is because only one copy of the purple color allele (B) is required for the phenotypic expression of purple flowers because it is dominant over the white color allele (b). A pea plant must be homozygous for the recessive allele in order to have a white color phenotype (bb), as the white blossom allele is recessive. Three out of four children will have purple flowers, while the fourth will have white flowers, as demonstrated by the Punnett square example (Figure 3.30).

Mendel proposed the Law of Segregation to describe how we may forecast the ratio of an offspring's genes to phenotypes. A parent will have two copies of a gene, each on a separate homologous chromosome, as was previously mentioned. According to the Law of Segregation, the two copies will be kept apart and given to their respective gametes. We now know that meiosis is the process that causes it.

Since babies are the result of the union of two gametes, they acquire one allele from each gamete for the majority of genes. The expected phenotypic ratios are easier to see when more offspring are generated, as in the case of pea plant breeding. Mendel's research on pea plants offers a straightforward framework for comprehending single-gene genetics. There are a few documented Mendelian features in humans, but many of the qualities anthropologists are interested in have more complex inheritance (for example, are influenced by many genes). Furthermore, a Mendelian pattern of inheritance is also seen in certain human disorders (Figure 3.31). Humans might find it more difficult to identify

Mendelian patterns since we do not have as many children as other organisms. It is nevertheless crucial to comprehend these ideas and be able to determine the likelihood that a child would exhibit a Mendelian phenotype.

Mendelian disorder	Gene	Mendelian disorder	Gene
Alpha Thalassemia	HBA1	Maple Syrup Urine Disease: Type 1A	BCKDHA
Androgen Insensitivity Syndrome	AR	Mitochondrial DNA Depletion Syndrome	TYMP
Bloom Syndrome	BLM	MTHFR Deficiency	MTHFR
Canavan Disease	ASPA	Oculocutaneous Albinism: Type 1	TYR
Cartilage-Hair Hypoplasia	RMRP	Oculocutaneous Albinism: Type 3	TYRP1
Cystic Fibrosis	CFTR	Persistent Mullerian Duct Syndrome: Type I	AMH
Familial Chloride Diarrhea	SLC26A3	Polycystic Kidney Disease	PKHD1
Fragile X Syndrome	FMR1	Sickle-cell anemia	HBB
Glucose-6-Phosphate Dehydrogenase Deficiency	G6PD	Spermatogenic failure	USP9Y
Hemophilia A	F8	Spinal Muscular Atrophy: SMN1 Linked	SMN1
Huntington disease	HTT	Tay-Sachs Disease	HEXA
Hurler Syndrome	IDUA	Wilson Disease	ATP7B

Figure 3.31 Mendelian inheritance patterns in human disorders.

The ABO Blood Group System is an illustration of Mendelian inheritance.

Karl Landsteiner, who discovered the ABO blood groups at the University of Vienna, published his findings in 1901. This resulted from his blood immunology investigations, when he mixed the blood of people with various blood cell types and saw a clotting (agglutination) reaction. While no agglutination will happen among people with the same blood type, the occurrence of agglutination indicates an immune reaction that is incompatible. The fact that this effort increased the survival rate of patients who got blood transfusions makes it evidently significant. Agglutinations from receiving blood transfusions from someone with a different blood type result in coagulated blood that is difficult to pass through blood arteries, which can be fatal. As a result, Landsteiner's explanation of the ABO blood type system earned him the Nobel Prize in 1930.

Red blood cells have proteins called blood cell surface antigens on their surface, and antibodies are "against" or "anti" to the antigens found in other blood types. Agglutination between blood types that are incompatible is thus caused by antibodies. Determining ABO compatibility between blood donors and receivers requires an understanding of how antigens and antibodies interact. Figure 3.32 shows blood cell antigens and plasma antibodies to help better understand blood phenotypes and ABO compatibility. Blood type A individuals contain anti-B antibodies that will attach to B antigens if they come into touch with them, as well as A antigens on the surface of their red blood cells. On the other hand, those with blood type B have antibodies against A and B antigens. Despite having both A and B antigens, people with blood type AB do not make antibodies against the ABO system. The absence of anti-A or anti-B antibodies does not imply that type AB is antibody-deficient. Despite having generic antigens, people with blood type O generate both anti-A and anti-B antibodies.

	Group A	Group B	Group AB	Group O
Red blood cell type	A	B	AB	O
Antibodies in Plasma	Anti-B	Anti-A	None	Anti-A and Anti-B
Antigens in Red Blood Cell	A antigen	B antigen	A and B antigens	None

Figure 3.32 shows the various ABO blood types together with the antigens and antibodies that correspond to them.

	A	B	O
A	AA	AB	AO
B	AB	BB	BO
O	AO	BO	OO

The various ABO blood allele combinations (A, B, and O) that result in ABO blood genotypes are shown in Figure 3.33.

The Mendelian inheritance pattern of the ABO allele system is displayed in a table in Figure 3.33. The B allele codes for the B antigen, while the A allele always codes for the A antigen because both alleles are dominant. In contrast to A and

B, the O allele codes for a nonfunctional antigen protein, meaning that O blood cells have no antigen on their cell surface. The O allele is regarded as recessive since two copies of it must be inherited, one from each parent, in order to have blood type O. Thus, a person with a heterozygous AO genotype has blood type A phenotype, while a person with a BO genotype has blood type B phenotype. Codominance, or the effect of both alleles on the phenotype, is also demonstrated by the ABO blood system. When a person with blood type AB inherits both the A and B alleles, their cell surface will have both A and B antigens.

The rhesus group antigen, or "Rh factor," is also present on the surface of red blood cells. Although red blood cells have a number of antigens that are not related to the ABO blood system, the Rh factor is the second most crucial antigen to take into account when assessing the compatibility of blood donors and recipients. When a pregnant woman and her unborn child have incompatible Rh factors, Rh antigens must also be taken into account. In these situations, a doctor can provide the appropriate medical care to avoid hemolytic illness, which occurs when the mother's antibodies destroy the newborn's red blood cells, and pregnancy difficulties.

A person may be Rh positive (having the Rh antigen) or Rh negative (without having the Rh antigen). The Rh factor is inherited separately from the ABO alleles and is regulated by a single gene. All blood types can therefore be classified as either negative (O-, A-, B-, AB-) or positive (O+, A+, B+, AB+).

Blood donors with O+ red blood cells can provide blood to recipients with A+, B+, AB+, and O+ blood types. O-persons are compatible with all blood cell types and are known as "universal donors" because they lack the AB or Rh antigens, while AB+ individuals are known as "universal recipients" because they lack antibodies against other blood types.

Mendelian Pedigree and Inheritance Patterns

By identifying whether a health condition is inherited and may need medical attention, a pedigree can be used to look into a family's medical history. Determining whether the ailment is dominant or Mendelian recessive can also be aided by a pedigree. A family with Huntington's disease, which has a Mendelian dominant pattern of inheritance, is shown in Figure 3.34. Males are shown as squares in a typical pedigree, while females are shown as circles. The square or circle is filled up as a solid color when a person has a particular condition. A child has a 50% chance of inheriting the faulty chromosome in a dominant condition, meaning that at least one parent will have the illness. As a result, every generation typically has dominating genetic conditions. Parents may unintentionally pass on Huntington's disease, a dominantly inherited disease, to their children because some people may not receive a diagnosis until later in life.

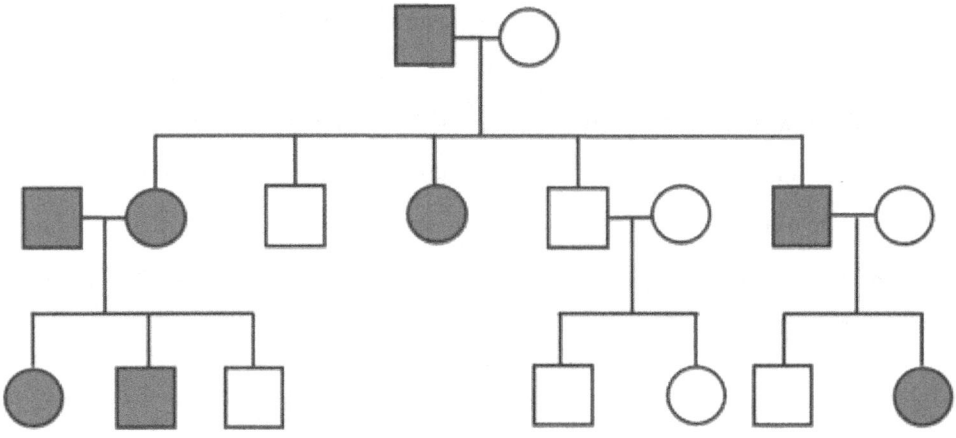

A three-generation pedigree illustrating Huntington's-like dominant Mendelian inheritance is shown in Figure 3.34.

Recessive medical disorders can skip generations since the likelihood of inheriting a recessive allele that causes the disease is lower. A family with a recessive cystic fibrosis mutation is shown in Figure 3.35. The likelihood of a parent passing on their chromosome to their offspring is 50% if they are heterozygous for the cystic fibrosis allele. When a child has a recessive disease, it indicates that both of their parents are heterozygous, or carriers, for that illness. Carriers of recessive disorders typically don't exhibit any significant health signs. Some people seek family planning services if there is a known medical history of a particular illness in their family.

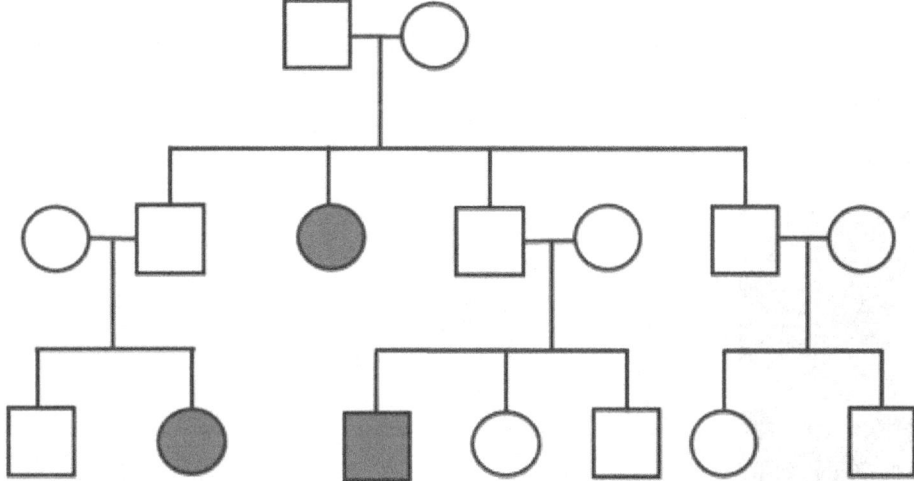

Figure 3.35: A three-generation pedigree showing a case of cystic fibrosis, a recessive Mendelian inheritance.

Additionally, pedigrees can assist in determining if a health problem is inherited in an autosomal or X-linked manner. There are 23 pairs of chromosomes, 22 of which are referred to as autosomes, as was previously mentioned. Autosomally related genetic illnesses are represented by the pedigree examples (Figure 3.34–35) that are supplied. This indicates that one of the chromosomes numbered 1 through 22 has the genes that cause the illness. Genes that cause disease may also be X-linked, meaning they are found on the X chromosome.

A family with a mother who carries the X-linked recessive disease Duchenne Muscular Dystrophy (DMD) is shown in Figure 3.36. Daughters and sons have a 50% probability of receiving the pathogenic DMD allele because the mother is a DMD carrier. Females will not get the disease because they have two X chromosomes, albeit in rare instances, female carriers may exhibit some disease signs. Males who inherit a copy of an X-linked pathogenic DMD allele, on the other hand, will usually have the disorder. Because males only have one X chromosome, they are more prone to X-linked disorders. Consequently, if a greater percentage of males in a lineage have the disease, this may indicate that the condition is X-linked recessive. Lastly, because the Y chromosome is smaller and contains fewer active (transcribed) genes than other chromosomes, Y-linked features are extremely uncommon.

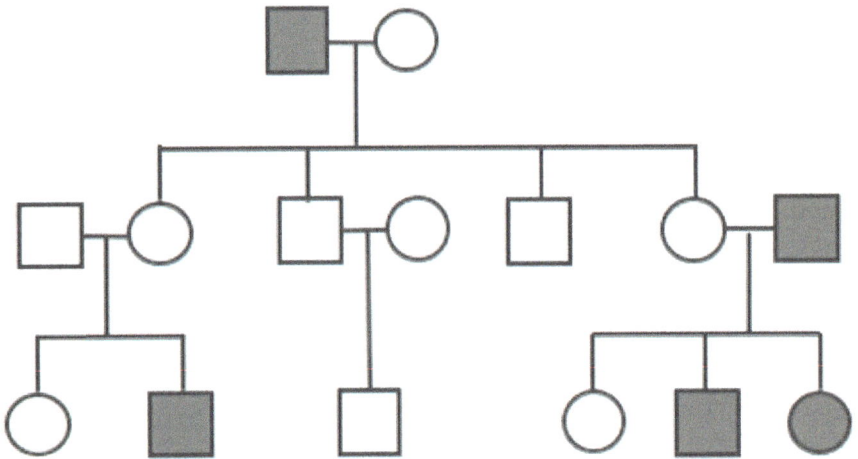

An illustration of X-linked Mendelian inheritance, such as Duchenne Muscular Dystrophy (DMD), is shown in Figure 3.36, which shows a three-generation pedigree.

Mendelian inheritance and its complexity

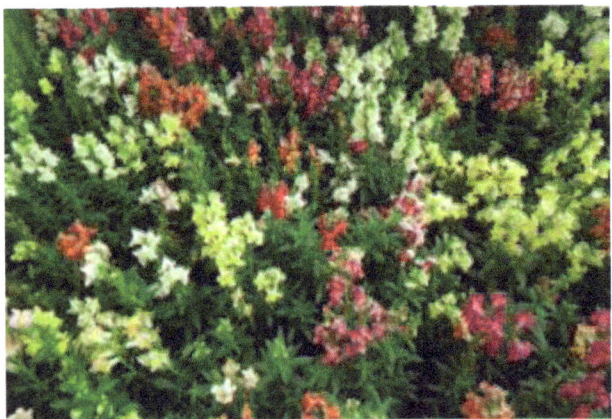

Snap dragons with varying genotypes exhibit phenotypic variations in bloom color (Figure 3.37).

Compared to our current understanding of genetic inheritance, pea plant trait genetics is quite straightforward. The link between alleles and phenotypic prediction is frequently more complex since the great majority of genetically regulated traits are neither absolutely dominant nor recessive. For instance, partial dominance refers to a heterozygous genotype that displays an intermediate phenotype of both alleles. The dominant flower color in snapdragons is red (R), whereas the recessive floral color is white (r). As a result, homozygous recessive rr is white while homozygous dominant RR is red. A pink blossom is produced by the heterozygote Rr, which is a mix of red and white due to the R allele's partial dominance (Figure 3.37).

The human enzyme β-hexosaminidase A (Hex A), which is encoded by the gene HEXA, is an example of incomplete dominance. A particular lipid-sugar compound (GM2 ganglioside) accumulates and damages nerve cells in the brain and spinal cord in patients with two malfunctioning HEXA alleles because they are unable to metabolize it. Tay-Sachs disease is the name of this disorder, which often manifests in newborns between the ages of three and six months. The majority of Tay-Sachs children do not survive past early childhood. Hex A activity is decreased in those who are heterozygous for one defective allele and the functional type HEXA allele. Nevertheless, carriers do not show any neurological abnormalities and seem healthy because there is still enough enzyme activity.

Additionally, some alleles and genes may be more penetrant than others. The percentage of people that possess a certain gene and exhibit the anticipated phenotype is known as penetration. Alleles are considered completely penetrant if they consistently result in the expected phenotype. Even if an individual has the alleles known to govern a characteristic or produce a disease, imperfect (or diminished) penetrance may prevent the occurrence of a predicted phenotype.

The genes BRCA1 and BRCA2 linked to cancer are a well-researched example of genetic penetrance. Breast and ovarian cancers may result from mutations in these genes that impact vital functions like DNA repair. A person who inherits a harmful allele does not necessarily develop cancer, even if BRCA1 and BRCA2 mutations exhibit an autosomal dominant pattern of inheritance. The chance of getting cancer can also be influenced by a number of environmental and lifestyle variables. In any case, it is frequently advised that those who are at risk undergo genetic testing if there is a family history of a particular cancer. Additionally, BRCA1/2 allele testing is now included in health reports provided by publicly accessible genetic testing companies.

POLYGENIC TRAITS

The great majority of human phenotypes are polygenic, whereas Mendelian features are often controlled by a single gene. Since the word "polygenic" implies "many genes," a polygenic characteristic is influenced by a large number of genes that combine to create the phenotype. Polygenic features include human phenotypes including weight, height, eye color, and hair color. A polygenic basis is also present in complex diseases, such as schizophrenia, Alzheimer's, and cardiovascular disorders.

One example of a polygenic trait is human hair color. The type and amount of a pigment called melanin, which is produced by a specific type of skin cell called melanocytes, determines the color of hair. Black, brown, blond, and red hair hues are determined by the amount and proportion of melanin pigments. A protein expressed on the surface of melanocytes and involved in the synthesis of eumelanin pigment is encoded by the well-studied gene MC1R. People who have two working copies of MC1R tend to be brown-haired. Pheomelanin production is more common in those with fewer functional copies of the MC1R gene, which causes blond or red hair. However, the penetrance of MC1R alleles varies, and research is constantly finding other genes that also affect hair color, such as TYR, TYRP1, SLC24A5, and

KITLG. People with oculocuteaneous albinism, a disorder caused by two non-functioning copies of the gene TYR, have pale skin, white hair, and light eyes because their melanocytes are unable to synthesize melanin.

Complex diseases are generally more common in humans than Mendelian diseases. Although complex diseases frequently lack a distinct pattern of heredity, they can also run in families. It's possible that geneticists are unaware of every gene linked to a particular complex illness. Complex diseases are impacted by a variety of environmental and lifestyle factors in addition to distinct gene combinations. Furthermore, it can be challenging to determine the relative contributions of each of these variables to a disease phenotype. Predicting medical risk is so frequently quite difficult. For example, one of the main causes of death worldwide is still cardiovascular diseases (CVDs). A number of genes, smoking, drug use, poor socioeconomic circumstances, high fat and sedentary lifestyles, and malnutrition during fetal development have all been connected to the development of CVDs. Human surroundings vary, and studies in public health, including human biology, can assist in identifying behaviors and risk factors linked to chronic illnesses. Some of these intricate relationships can also be clarified by extensive genetic research.

EPIGENETICS AND GENOMICS

The entirety of an organism's genetic material is called its genome. This comprises mtDNA and 46 chromosomes in humans. There are both coding and noncoding sections in the human genome, which has about three billion base pairs of DNA. According to current estimates, there are between 20,000 and 25,000 protein-coding genes in the human genome, with hundreds to thousands of genes found on each chromosome. The significance of epigenetics—alterations in gene expression that do not alter the underlying DNA sequence—has come to light as our understanding of heredity has grown. Deciphering gene regulation, which entails intricate relationships between DNA, RNA, proteins, and the environment, also depends heavily on epigenetics research.

Genomics

The great majority of the human genome is noncoding, which means that it lacks the instructions necessary to produce an RNA or protein. Since these large portions of the genome were believed to be unimportant and non-functional, noncoding DNA was previously known as "junk DNA." Nonetheless, ongoing advancements in DNA sequencing technology as well as international scientific partnerships and consortia have helped us better grasp how the genome works. We have since learned that many of these noncoding DNA sequences are involved in dynamic genetic regulation mechanisms thanks to these technical advancements and collaborations.

Gene mapping, genotyping (identifying the alleles present), and genomic evolution, structure, and function are the main topics of the broad discipline of molecular biology known as genomics. According to evolutionary genomics, humans and chimpanzees have a substantial amount of DNA in common (about 98.8%). Considering the behavioral distinctions between chimps and humans, a 1.2% DNA sequence difference appears unexpected. Finding out how noncoding genomic areas affect how specific genes are switched "on" and "off" (i.e., regulated) is the focus of much genomics research. Therefore, it is thought that the physical variations between humans and chimpanzees are mostly caused by regulatory changes in noncoding genetic areas (such as promoters), even if their DNA sequences are identical.

New medicines and individualized treatments for a variety of diseases may result from a deeper comprehension of genetic regulatory factors. For instance, a pathogenic gene's otherwise detrimental consequences can be avoided by focusing on its regulatory region to "turn off" its expression. These molecular targeting strategies can be tailored to a person's genetic composition. Genome-wide association studies (GWAS), which usually include a large amount of computer work, aim to identify the genes associated with complex traits and disorders. This is due to the fact that GWAS occasionally involve thousands of people and that millions of DNA sequences need to be examined. The majority of large-scale genomics research conducted in the early years of the field exclusively comprised patients and participants from North America, Europe, and East Asia. Increasing ethnic diversity in genetic studies and databases is currently a focus of research. This will lead to the identification of more rare disease-causing alleles and an improvement in the accuracy of individual disease risk across all human groups.

The study of epigenetics

Your body's cells all contain identical copies of DNA. For instance, a skin cell on your arm and a brain neuron share the same DNA code. These cells are regarded as specialized even though they share the same genetic makeup. Different subsets of genes are turned "on" and "off" inside the various cell types, which explains why all of the body's cells have the same DNA but differ in morphology and function. A more accurate interpretation is that various cell types have diverse gene expression patterns. A special subset of genes is active in neuronal cells, enabling them to develop axons for message transmission and reception. Skin cells and other non-neuronal cell types will not have this collection of genes. The study of how these genes are controlled by means that do not alter the underlying DNA sequence is known as epigenetics. A well-known instance of epigenetic regulation is described in Special Topics: Epigenetics and X Chromosome Inactivation.

DNA methylation and histone modifications are examples of epigenetic processes that take place on, above, or close to DNA. The word epi means "on, above, or near." DNA methylation occurs when a methyl group (—CH_3) is added to DNA (Figure 3.38). Chromatin is believed to become more compact due to DNA methylation and other changes caused to the histones that encircle DNA. Because transcription factors and RNA polymerases cannot access this DNA, genes cannot be activated (transcribed). In contrast, other histone changes relax chromatin, allowing transcription factors to reach genes.

It is crucial to remember that environmental influences can change histone modifications and DNA methylation, and that these changes can be inherited from one generation to the next. For instance, after stressful events (such as starvation, natural catastrophes, etc.), an individual's epigenetic profile may change, and the following generation may inherit these regulatory alterations. Furthermore, as we age, our profile of epigenetic expression shifts. For instance, throughout time, some regions of our genome become "hyper" or "hypo" methylation. Additionally, the epigenetic profiles of identical twins diverge more with age. The significance of all these genome-wide epigenetic alterations is still being uncovered by researchers. Researchers have also found that variations in epigenetic alterations can modify how genes are expressed, which can lead to diseases. It's also critical to remember that epigenetic modifications are easily reversible, in contrast to DNA mutations, which alter the nucleotide sequence irreversibly. Nowadays, a lot of study focuses on how medications can treat diseases like cancer by changing or modulating histone modifications and DNA methylation alterations.

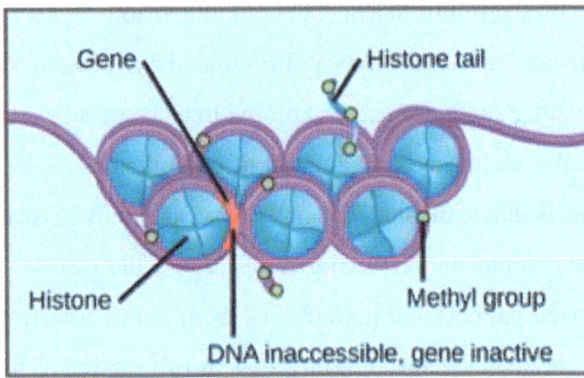
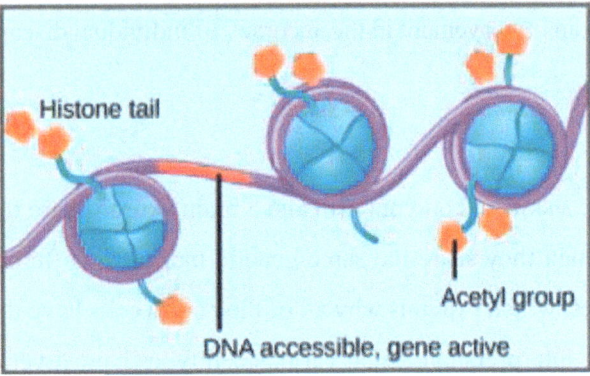

Different epigenetic changes of the histone tail that might tighten (top) or relax (bottom) the DNA chromatin are shown in Figure 3.38.

SPECIAL TOPIC: X CHROMOSOME INACTIVATION AND EPIGENETICS

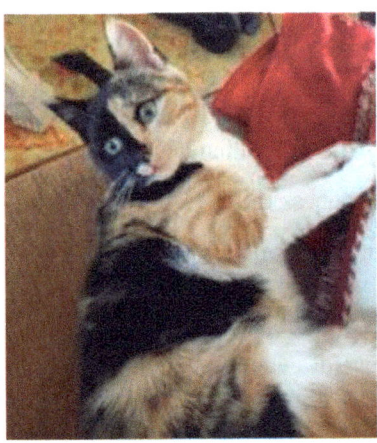

Figure 3.39 X chromosome inactivation during development results in a colorful coat pattern.

Based on her research and other studies conducted at the time, British geneticist Mary Lyon proposed the Lyon hypothesis, which states that X chromosomes can be inactivated. One X chromosome from each parent is inherited by females. Even though men only have one functional X chromosome, this does not imply that women have more active genes than men. Female mammals have one functioning X chromosome because one of their X chromosomes is randomly inactivated during genetic embryonic development. In females, epigenetic processes including DNA methylation and histone alterations are responsible for the inactivation of the X chromosome. Recent research has examined the function of Xinactive specific transcript (XIST), a lengthy noncoding RNA that plays a major role in the random silencing of one of the X chromosomes. In order to inactivate one X chromosome, the expression of XIST RNA is triggered by the presence of two X chromosomes. The maternal X chromosome may be active in some cells, whereas the paternal X chromosome may be active in others. Calico and tortoiseshell cats readily exhibit this phenomena (Figure 3.39). In cats, the X chromosome contains the gene that determines coat color. The distinct coat patterning is caused by groups of cells that express black or orange due to random inactivation of the X chromosome during early embryonic development. As a result, calico cats are usually female.

TESTING GENETIC

In the United States, newborn screening for genetic illnesses has been available for more than 50 years to support public health initiatives. Confirming a diagnosis of phenylketonuria (PKU) in infants—a condition that can be readily treated with dietary modifications—was one of the earliest genetic tests that were available. The genes that are included on newborn screening panels are now determined by each state, and some even have initiatives to assist with infant medical follow-ups.

Testing for a few thousand different genes is now available in hundreds of labs, which can help guide medical decisions for both adults and newborns. Technology breakthroughs and patient cost reductions are what have enabled this sector. Furthermore, genetic testing is now openly accessible to everyone without the help of medical experts.

Sanger sequencing and the Polymerase Chain Reaction (PCR)

The polymerase chain reaction (PCR) was one of the most significant innovations in the science of genetics. The concentration needs to reach specific levels in order for scientists to see and, consequently, examine DNA. Millions of copies of DNA can be amplified from a very small amount of template DNA thanks to PCR, which was created by Kary Mullis in 1985 (Figure 3.40). For instance, it is possible to amp up and test for a DNA match from a trace amount of DNA found at a crime scene. Additionally, as aDNA usually degrades, ancient genomes can be rebuilt by amplifying the few DNA molecules that remain. Similar biochemical processes that occur in our own cells during DNA replication are used in the PCR experiment.

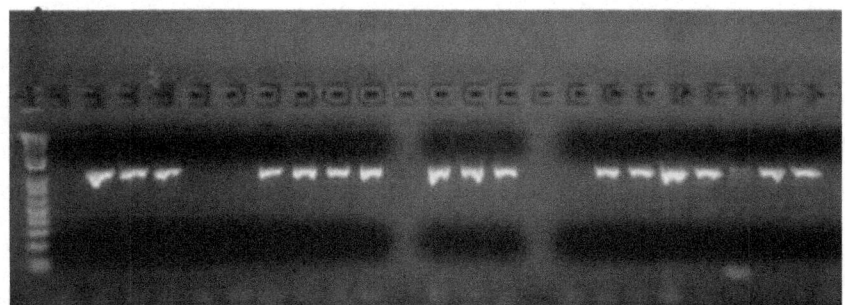

After PCR amplification, DNA is visualized using gel electrophoresis (Figure 3.40).

Fluorescent labeling in Sanger sequencing allows PCR sequences to be examined at the nucleotide level. This assay allows for the detection of various alleles and genetic alterations in DNA. A person who is heterozygous for a single nucleotide allele is depicted in Figure 3.41. These techniques are still widely employed in conjunction with more sophisticated genomic technologies.

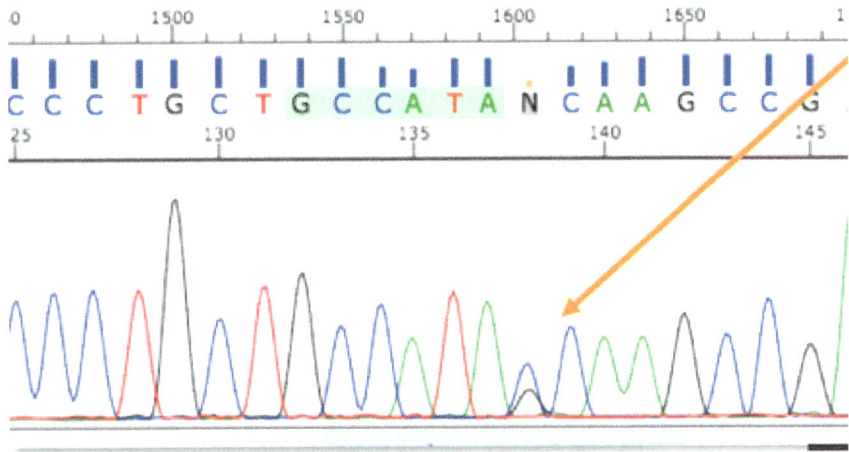

A heterozygous DNA nucleotide is displayed in Figure 3.41, which displays the results of Sanger sequencing.

Clinical Testing and Genetic Biotechnology

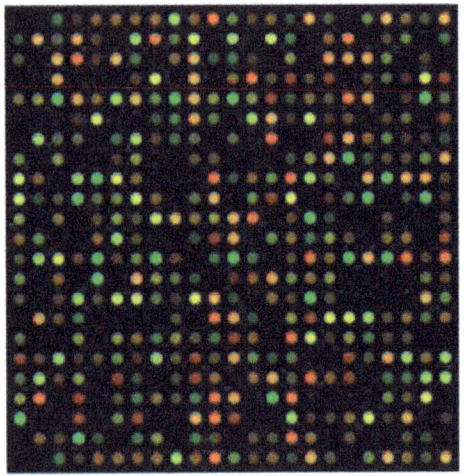

Figure 3.42: A microarray chip with fluorescently labeled probes that identify homozygous and heterozygous nucleotides across the genome by hybridizing with DNA.

Innovations in genetics are revolutionizing the medical field. However, there is frequently a learning curve for patients, the general public, and medical professionals due to the various forms of technology and the outcomes of these tests. Microarray technology has been around for a while and is used to genotype (or "screen") DNA samples for particular alleles (Figure 3.42). These days, hundreds of alleles that are known to be linked to different diseases can be found on microarray chips. Only when a DNA sample is "positive" for that specific allele and a fluorescent signal is released, which can be further examined, can the microarray chip bond with it.

Whole genome sequencing may be suggested by a physician if a patient is suspected of having a rare genetic disorder that is difficult to detect or if the diagnosis is completely unknown. A more recent technique, next-generation sequencing (NGS), may screen the entire genome by examining millions of sequences in a single machine run (Figure 3.43).

Nonetheless, a substantial amount of data and information can be obtained by sequencing the complete genome. Therefore, just a limited portion of the genome known to have pathogenic disease-causing mutations is usually included in clinical NGS genetic testing.

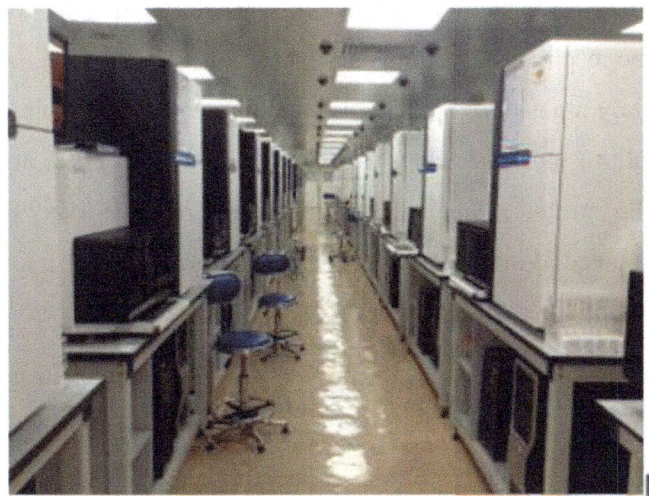

Figure 3.43: Machines for next-generation sequencing.

A variety of clinical genetics tests, such as those for embryo genetic screening and in vitro fertilization (IVF), are available to help individuals make health and family planning decisions based on medical knowledge. All clinical laboratories must be continuously regulated in order to guarantee accuracy. All human laboratory testing centers are required to adhere to the Clinical Laboratory Improvement Amendments (CLIA), which are federal regulations in the United States. Access to genetic counselors, who possess specific education and experience in medical genetics and counseling, is a significant advantage offered by certain clinical genetic testing companies. To determine whether there is a chance of a disease being passed on to a child, both spouses are often tested. Counselors utilize their expertise to help physicians and patients understand the results of genetic testing and assess their risk for hereditary illnesses. Additionally, genetic counselors help patients make important medical decisions by offering guidance and support.

Direct Genetic Testing to Consumers (DTC)

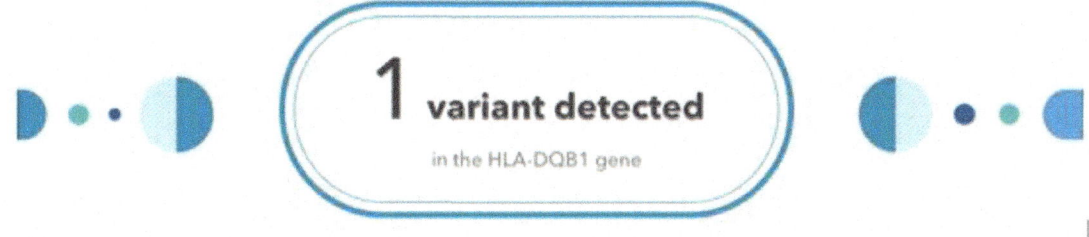

A positive result for a genetic allele linked to a higher risk of celiac disease is shown in Figure 3.44.

Direct-to-consumer (DTC) genetic testing refers to genetic testing that is carried out without the supervision of medical personnel. Businesses that provide the general public with reasonably priced genome sequencing solutions are becoming more and more common. The marketing campaigns of these companies are usually centered around the idea of "personal empowerment," which can be attained by "knowing more about your DNA." For instance, if you are found to have a slightly elevated risk of celiac disease (Figure 3.44), you might be inspired to change your diet by cutting out gluten. A known harmful BRCA1 or BRCA2 allele could also be detected by a positive test. In this situation, you might wish to follow up with more testing from a medical facility, which could result in decisions that change your life. There are additional products that use DNA sequencing for amusement. For instance, you can find out if you are more likely to prefer Pinots as your favorite wine by having your "Vinome" examined. Furthermore, it is possible to genotype a person and their partner in order to anticipate the physical traits that their unborn child may inherit.

DTC testing usually has less stringent requirements and no genetic counselor services. Some concerns have resulted from this, such as business genetic goods that offer health information. DTC health testing was originally made available on the market by 23andMe, and in 2013, the U.S. The FDA (Food and Drug Administration) stepped in. 23andMe obtained authorized to provide testing on a few medically linked genes after working to comply with FDA rules. A genetic risk report for "Late-Onset Alzheimer's Disease" was made available by 23andMe in 2017. Customers may receive outcomes from such products that they may not completely understand, which has led to criticism. As a result, people may experience more stress (often referred to as the "burden of knowing") and may needless medical intervention. To solve this problem, 23andMe now requires users to finish interactive learning sessions and disclaimers before they can view specific genotyping results. Nonetheless, people who have tested positive for an allele that causes the condition have also been successful in getting medical attention. There is still discussion and research surrounding the possible risks and suggested advantages of DTC testing.

European		**91.6%**
• British & Irish		32.9%
United Kingdom		
• Scandinavian		5.9%
• Iberian		4.3%
• French & German		1.6%
Netherlands		
• Ashkenazi Jewish		0.5%
• Broadly Northwestern European		34.6%
• Broadly Southern European		6.0%
• Broadly European		5.8%
East Asian & Native American		**7.8%**
• Native American		6.4%
Mexico		
We predict you had ancestors that lived in Mexico within the last 200 years.		
• Broadly East Asian		0.1%
• Broadly East Asian & Native American		1.4%
South Asian		**0.2%**
• Broadly South Asian		0.2%
Sub-Saharan African		**0.1%**
• West African		0.1%
Unassigned		**0.4%**

An illustration of ancestry percentage results given to clients is shown in Figure 3.45.

Additionally, many people use ancestry percentage testing (Figure 3.45). Consumers are genotyped, and their alleles are allocated to various global groupings. However, others have questioned the scientific value and possible risks of ancestry percentage tests. For instance, populations may be defined differently by testing companies, and the majority of alleles examined are not unique to any one population. The allele may have originated in a separate cultural group or location that existed before the country of Ireland was formed, if it is attributed to the "Irish" people. To put it another way, genetic variance frequently predates the population's origins and the region's geographical labels that genetic testing businesses employ. Another criticism is that biological ties are not necessary for defining an individual's identity. People can also use the internet to locate and interact with people who share parts of their DNA, which can have both beneficial and bad effects. The fact that law enforcement is now creating forensic methods that use DTC genomic database mining to find people connected to crimes is another intriguing factor to take into account. Notwithstanding these different factors, millions of people worldwide have now "unlocked the secrets" of their DNA, and the multibillion-dollar genomics sector is only expected to rise.

DNA gives our cells instructions, which leads to the production and control of proteins, as you have seen in this chapter. To comprehend how the evolutionary process operates and how humans differ from one another, it is essential to comprehend these basic mechanisms. Additionally, fresh anthropological insights on our biological links to other extinct and current primates have been made possible by the development of genetic technology, such as genomics, epigenetics, and ancient DNA research. In the upcoming chapters, several of these genetic discoveries will be discussed.

Review Questions

- Why does DNA replication occur? Give a brief explanation of the steps involved in DNA replication. When do mutations in DNA occur? What causes phenotypic variety, or distinct phenotypes of the same physical characteristic, as a result of this?
- Describe sister chromatids and homologous chromosomes in your own terms. What are meiosis and mitosis's main distinctions?
- Identify whether the pedigree diagram below shows an X-linked recessive, autosomal dominant, or autosomal recessive pattern of inheritance. To assist you, you should write the genotype (AA, Aa, or aa) above each square (keep in mind that there may occasionally be two alternative solutions for a square's genotype). Additionally, could you please explain your reasoning for choosing that specific inheritance pattern?

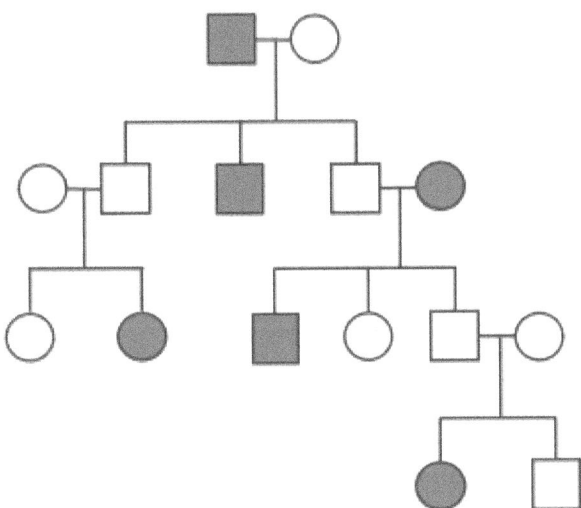

- Figure 3.46
- To convert the DNA template sequence GTAAAGGTGCTGGCCATC into mRNA, apply base pairing principles. Next, translate the sequence using the protein codon table (Figure 3.25). Describe the importance of the first and last codons or proteins in the sequence in relation to transcription.
- What advantages do you believe direct-to-consumer (DTC) genetic testing offers? What are the disadvantages and/or more significant moral issues? Do you believe that advantages outweigh drawbacks?

- Suppose you send a DNA sample to a genetic testing company, and they identify an allele linked to late-onset Alzheimer's disease among the many disorders they test for. The choice to view or not view your Alzheimer's result is up to you. Why do you do what you do?

Important Words

Adenosine Triphosphate (ATP): Cellular functions are powered by adenosine triphosphate (ATP), a high-energy substance generated by mitochondria.

Allele: An allele is a non-identical DNA sequence that codes for the same trait but results in a distinct phenotype. It can be located in the same gene position on a homologous chromosome, or gene copy.

Protein is made up of organic compounds called **amino acids**. Every one of the twenty distinct amino acids possesses a distinct chemical characteristic. Proteins are similarly made up of chains of amino acids.

Ancient DNA, or aDNA:, is DNA extracted from organic remnants that are frequently hundreds to thousands of years old. Also, exposure to environmental factors like heat, acidity, and humidity usually causes aDNA to deteriorate, or become damaged.

A cell that has an unusually high number of chromosomes is called **aneuploid**. Chromosomes may be gained or lost during meiotic or mitotic division.

Antibodies are immune-related proteins that have the ability to recognize and attach to infections and other foreign substances in the blood.

Apoptosis: A set of molecular processes that trigger cell death. Although cancer cells can evade apoptosis, it can be triggered when a cell misses checkpoints during the cell cycle.

Autosomal: Describes an inheritance type in which an allele is found on an autosome.

Base pairs: are chemical bonds formed between nucleotides, such as those between adenine (A) and uracil (U) in RNA or cytosine (C) and guanine (G) in DNA.

Carbohydrates: Carbon and hydrogen atoms make up molecules known as carbohydrates, which can be broken down to release energy.

Carrier: A carrier is a person who carries a heterozygous genotype, which is commonly linked to a disease.

Cell cycle: A cycle that a cell goes through with checkpoints in between phases to make sure that cell division and DNA replication run smoothly.

Cell Surface Antigen: A protein present on the surface of red blood cells is known as a cell surface antigen.

Centromere: A structural characteristic that produces two distinct arm lengths and is referred to as the "center" of a chromosome. The term also describes the area where microtubules bind during meiosis and mitosis.

Chromatin: DNA encircled by histone complexes is called chromatin. Chromatin transforms into a condensed chromosome during cell division.

Chromosome: The DNA molecule known as a chromosome is encircled by protein complexes, such as histones.

Codominance: A genotype's phenotype reflects the effects of both alleles.

Codons: Three DNA nucleotides that together code for a protein are called codons.

Complex diseases: A group of polygenic illnesses that are also impacted by lifestyle and environmental variables.

Cytoplasm: The "jelly-like" matrix that houses many organelles and other cellular substances is called cytoplasm.

Detrimental: A mutation that makes an organism more prone to illness is considered detrimental.

Deoxyribonucleic acid (DNA): A molecule called deoxyribonucleic acid (DNA) contains the genetic information that parents pass on to their children. One way to characterize DNA is as a "double helix." It has a sugar-phosphate backbone and two chains of nucleotides joined by hydrogen bonds.

Diploid: A cell or organism that has two sets of chromosomes is said to be diploid.

DNA methylation: When methyl groups attach to DNA, they change a gene's transcriptional activity by making it "on" or "off."

DNA polymerase: During DNA replication, the enzyme DNA polymerase adds nucleotides to already-existing nucleic acid strands. The processivity of certain enzymes (such as DNA replication) allows for their differentiation.

DNA replication is the process by which DNA is duplicated and doubled within cells.

DNA sequence: The nucleotide base order is known as the DNA sequence. A DNA sequence may be brief, lengthy, or indicative of an organism's genome or all of its chromosomes.

Dominant: An allele is said to be dominant if only one copy is needed for the phenotype to manifest.

Elongation: The process by which DNA polymerases help create new DNA from template strands.

Enzymes: Proteins called enzymes are in charge of catalyzing, or speeding up, a variety of metabolic processes within cells.

Epigenetic profile: The methylation pattern across a genome, or the genes (and other genomic locations) that are methylated and unmethylated, is known as the epigenetic profile.

Epigenetics: Changes in gene expression that do not alter the underlying DNA sequence are known as epigenetics. Histone modifications and DNA methylation are frequently involved in these alterations. These modifications can be undone and passed down to the following generation.

Euchromatin: The nucleus contains loosely wound chromosomes that are available for DNA regulatory processing.

Eukaryotes: are single- or multicellular organisms that have a unique nucleus and membranes enclosing each organelle.

Exon: A gene's protein-coding section.

Gametes: During sexual reproduction, haploid cells known as an egg and sperm will unite to form a diploid organism.

Gene: A gene is a section of DNA that includes different regulatory (like a promoter) and noncoding (like introns) sections in addition to protein-coding information.

Genetic recombination: During meiosis I, a biological process known as genetic recombination takes place where sister chromatids on distinct chromosomes physically exchange genetic information and homologous chromosomes couple up.

Genome: An organism's whole genetic makeup.

Genotype: Two alleles that code for or are connected to the same gene make up a genotype.

Genotyping: is a molecular technique used to find new alleles or check for the presence of specific ones.

Haploid: A cell or creature that has one set of chromosomes is said to be haploid (n = 23).

Helicase: A protein called helicase is responsible for rupturing the hydrogen bonds that bind double-stranded DNA.

Heterozygous: A genotype with two distinct alleles is called heterozygous.

Histones: are proteins that DNA clings to in order to help organize DNA in the nucleus.

Homologous: A matching pair of chromosomes in which one is inherited from the mother and the other from the father is known as homologous chromosomes.

Homozygous: A genotype with two identical alleles is called homozygous.

Heterozygous: A heterozygous genotype that results in a phenotype that combines the traits of both alleles is known as incomplete dominance.

Initiation: The recruitment of proteins to split DNA strands and start DNA replication is known as initiation.

Interphase: The stage of the cell cycle before division, when a rise in metabolic demand permits DNA replication and cell doubling.

Introns: DNA segments known as introns are responsible for not coding for proteins.

Karyotyping: The process of counting chromosomes in a cell under a microscope.

Lagging strand: The DNA template strand opposite the leading strand is known as the lagging strand. As a result, Okazaki fragments are produced when DNA replication progresses irregularly.

Leading strand: The DNA template strand that replicates constantly is known as the leading strand.

Lipids: are fatty acid molecules that have a number of functions in cells, such as structure, signaling, and energy storage.

Meiosis: Gametes divide through a process called meiosis. Four haploid daughter cells are produced at the completion of meiosis.

Mendelian genetics: A term used to describe phenotypic characteristics that are regulated by a single gene.

Messenger RNA (mRNA): Transcribed from DNA, messenger RNA (mRNA) is an RNA molecule. A ribosome "reads" its tri-nucleotide codons to create a protein.

Microarray technology: A method of genotyping that makes use of a microarray chip, which is a solid surface containing thousands of short nucleotide sequences that may be used to probe genomic DNA.

Microbiome: The aggregate genomes of the population of microorganisms that inhabit human bodies are referred to as the microbiome.

Mitochondrial DNA (mtDNA): A circular DNA segment that is inherited from the mother and found in mitochondria.

Mitochondria: The specialized cellular organelle known as the mitochondria is where energy is produced. Additionally, it possesses its own genome (mtDNA).

Mitosis: The process by which somatic cells divide is called mitosis. Two diploid daughter cells are produced at the completion of mitosis.

Mutation: During replication, a nucleotide sequence deviation from the template DNA strand may take place. Recombination can also result in mutations.

Next-generation sequencing: is a genotyping technique that uses a single DNA sample to create millions of nucleotide sequences, which are subsequently read by a sequencing machine. It necessitates substantial program-based applications and can be used to analyze individual portions or entire genomes.

Nuclear envelope: The double-layered membrane that surrounds the nucleus is known as the nuclear envelope.

Nucleic acid: A complex structure that contains genetic information about a living thing, such as DNA or RNA, is called a nucleic acid.

Nucleic: DNA (A, T, C, and G) and RNA (A, U, C, and G) are examples of nucleotides, which are the fundamental structural building blocks of nucleic acids.

Nucleus: The double-membrane cellular organelle known as the nucleus aids in the regulation of nuclear activity and DNA protection.

Okazaki fragments: Short DNA strands produced by DNA replication on the lagging strand are known as Okazaki fragments. In the 1960s, Reiji and Tsuneko Okazaki made the discovery.

Organelle: A cell's internal structure that carries out certain functions that are vital to the cell. Organelles come in various varieties, each with a unique function.

Pathogenic: An allele, or genetic mutation, that causes a disease with a detrimental phenotypic consequence.

Penetrance: The percentage of times a predicted trait is produced by having an allele. Different alleles have varying levels of penetrantness.

Phenotype: A trait's outward manifestation.

Phospholipid bilayer: is a barrier made up of two layers of lipids with a hydrophilic (loving water) head and a hydrophobic (repelling water) tail.

Polygenic trait: A phenotype that is regulated by two or more genes is called a polygenic trait.

Polymerase chain reaction (PCR): A molecular biology technique called polymerase chain reaction (PCR) may replicate genomic DNA segments. Millions of copies are created using a tiny amount of DNA as a starting template.

Primer: is a brief nucleotide sequence that binds DNA to initiate the PCR or DNA replication process.

Prokaryotes: are single-celled organisms that lack membrane-enclosed organelles and a nucleus.

Promoter: The part of a gene that starts transcription is called the promoter. The transcriptional activity of a gene can be altered by the binding of transcription factors and DNA methylation at a promoter region.

Protein: A three-dimensional chain of amino acids that enables a cell to perform a number of functions.

Protein synthesis: is a multi-step process in which RNA machinery reads a DNA template to string amino acids together.

Recessive: A recessive allele is one whose effects are typically not observed unless an individual's genotype has two copies of the allele.

Ribonucleic acid (RNA): Single-stranded nucleic acid molecules are called ribonucleic acid (RNA). Cells contain many RNAs that carry out a range of tasks, including protein production and cell signaling.

Ribosomal RNA (rRNA): A molecule attached to ribosomes, ribosomal RNA (rRNA) is necessary for the proper assembly of amino acids into proteins.

Ribosome: An organelle in the cytoplasm or endoplasmic reticulum of a cell is called a ribosome. It is in charge of reading protein assemblage and mRNA.

RNA polymerase: An enzyme called RNA polymerase catalyzes the conversion of a DNA template into RNA.

Sanger-sequencing: A technique that visualizes DNA (PCR fragments) at the nucleotide level by using fluorescently labeled nucleotides.

Semi-conservative replication: DNA replication that creates new DNA from an existing DNA template strand is known as semi-conservative replication.

Sequencing: is a molecular laboratory technique that generates nucleotide base order, or sequences.

Sister chromatids: The chromosome produces sister chromatids during DNA replication. Sister chromatids are separated during cell division to create two new cells. Sister chromatids are also where genetic recombination occurs during meiosis.

Somatic cells: are diploid cells that make up bodily tissues and go through mitosis to keep and repair them.

Splicing: The procedure that produces mature mRNAs is called splicing. Exons are linked together and introns are cut off (spliced).

Sugar-phosphate backbone: One of DNA's biological structural elements is the sugar-phosphate backbone. Phosphate molecules and deoxyribose sugars make up the "backbone."

Telomere: After each round of cell division, the telomere—a composite structure at the ends of chromosomes—helps shield them from deterioration.

Termination: When a DNA sequence "stop" codon is discovered, DNA replication activity stops.

Tissue: A collection of cells with similar morphologies and functions.

Transcription: The process of copying DNA nucleotides (inside a gene) to create a messenger RNA molecule is called transcription.

Transcription factors: are proteins that attach to the promoter or other regulatory areas of genes to change their transcriptional activity, so turning them "on" or "off."

Transfer RNA (tRNA): An RNA molecule involved in translation is called transfer RNA (tRNA). Amino acids are transported to a ribosome by transfer RNA from the cytoplasm of the cell.

Translation: is the process via which amino acids are "chained together" to make proteins and messenger RNA codons are read.

X-linked: The term "X-linked" describes an inheritance pattern in which the allele is found on either the X or Y chromosome.

What is Biochemistry?

Biochemistry is the scientific field that studies all biological processes, including coordination and control within living things.

In the year 1930, the father of biochemistry, Carl Neuberg, first used this word. This area of study examines the chemical makeup of living things by fusing chemistry and biology. The biochemists do research in a variety of labs by studying the chemical reactions and combinations that are involved in processes such as growth, metabolism, inheritance, and reproduction.

Both molecular and cell biology are covered in great detail in Introduction to Biochemistry. It is pertinent to molecular anatomy, which is the study of molecules that comprise the structure of cells and organs. It explains the reactions that carbon compounds go through in living things. Additionally, it explains molecular physiology, which is the study of how molecules fulfill the needs of cells and organs.

Its primary focus is on the structure and activities of biomolecules, including lipids, proteins, carbohydrates, and acids. For this reason, it is also known as molecular biology.

Five justifications for studying biochemistry

1. **Expertise**

Whether you wish to work in industry or continue in education and research in a particular subject, biochemistry is versatile and may be used to many different fields and specializations. The University of Strathclyde allows you to further customize your biochemistry degree by allowing you to combine biochemistry with other biomolecular science courses. This allows you to explore your interests and areas of specialization. Immunology, microbiology, and pharmacology are among the combined programs.

2. Opportunities for careers

If you are currently uncertain about your future, biochemistry is the ideal major to pursue because it can lead to a wide variety of related occupations. Among many other professions, you could work in forensics, product development, healthcare, or a research lab. Since you are studying the fundamentals of life by selecting biochemistry, your alternatives are virtually limitless. This is bolstered at Strathclyde by a robust research foundation, connections with business, the NHS, and international partners, all of which helped the program rank among the top 5 in the UK for Biological Sciences.

3. Skills that are transferable

You need more than just your degree to land a job after graduation; you also need transferable abilities that are relevant to the position you're seeking for. You will acquire problem-solving, data analysis, process development, and project management abilities in biochemistry, which are essential for any field you decide to pursue. When you're ready to start looking for a job, you can apply to a greater number of positions. In addition to working in labs, many biochemistry graduates go on to pursue careers in business, education, or finance.

4. Creativity

Studying biochemistry entails experimenting and developing fresh perspectives on how systems function. This is a useful life and professional skill that will improve your chances of landing a job. Developing a fresh perspective can open you special chances. Whether it's medical drug research, genome sequencing, food and agricultural developments, or something else entirely, the process of testing hypotheses will equip you to make advancements in your chosen profession.

5. Recognize the molecular underpinnings of life

Finding answers to the world's numerous problems may depend on our ability to comprehend life and the processes that make it up. Selecting biochemistry will equip you with the knowledge and skills need to better comprehend the world and make improvements.

Biochemistry

Have you ever seen how the human body goes through chemical processes or reactions? How do metabolic processes occur? Yes, "Biochemistry" will teach you about all of these living processes.

Biochemistry's Branches

This subsection enumerates the main fields of biochemistry.

Molecular Biology

Another name for it is the foundations of biochemistry. It focuses on the study of how living systems work. This branch of biology describes how DNA, proteins, and RNA interact as well as how they are synthesized.

The study of cells

The structure and operations of cells in living things are the subject of cell biology. Another name for it is cytology. Instead of concentrating on prokaryotes, which will be the subject of microbiology, cell biology mainly studies the signaling pathways and cells of eukaryotic species.

The metabolism

One of the most significant processes occurring in all living organisms is metabolism. It is simply the changes or sequence of actions that take place in the human body when food is transformed into energy. The digesting process is one instance of metabolism.

Genetics

The study of genes, their variations, and the traits of heredity in living things is the focus of the biochemistry field of genetics.

Molecular chemistry, genetic engineering, endocrinology, pharmaceuticals, neurochemistry, nutrition, environmental, photosynthesis, toxicology, biotechnology, animal and plant biochemistry, and more are among the various subfields.

The Significance of Biochemistry

The following ideas require an understanding of biochemistry.

- The chemical reactions that convert dietary components into chemicals that define a species' cells.
- Enzymes' catalytic activities.
- Making use of the potential energy that is produced when food is oxidized for the several energy-demanding functions of the living cell.
- The characteristics and composition of the materials that make up tissues and cells.
- To address basic issues in biology and medicine.

What is Immunology?

One of the most significant areas of the biological and medical sciences is immunology, which is the study of the immune system. Through a number of defense mechanisms, the immune system keeps us safe from illness. Diseases including cancer, allergies, and autoimmune diseases can arise from the immune system not working properly. Additionally, it is increasingly evident that immune responses play a role in the emergence of other prevalent disorders that are not typically thought of as immunologic, such as cardiovascular, metabolic, and neurodegenerative diseases like Alzheimer's.

What makes immunology significant?

Immunology has changed the face of modern medicine since Edward Jenner's groundbreaking work in the 18th century led to the development of vaccination in its modern form, which has probably saved more lives than any other medical advancement. Other scientific advances in the 19th and 20th centuries included the identification of blood groups, safe organ transplantation, and the now-commonplace use of monoclonal antibodies in science and medicine. With continuous research efforts in immunotherapy, autoimmune illnesses, and vaccines for emerging viruses like Ebola, immunological research keeps expanding our understanding of how to address serious health conditions. In addition to being crucial for clinical and commercial applications, expanding our knowledge of basic immunology has made it easier to develop novel diagnostics and treatments for a variety of illnesses. In addition to the aforementioned, immunological research has produced vitally significant research tools and procedures, like flow cytometry and antibody technology, in conjunction with developing technology.

An immunologist: what is it?

A scientist and/or clinician with expertise in immunology is known as an immunologist. Numerous immunologists are employed in research-focused labs in both the business sector (such as the pharmaceutical industry) and academia. Other immunologists, often known as "clinical immunologists," are medical professionals who specialize in the diagnosis and treatment of immune system disorders such allergies and autoimmune illnesses.

The immune system

The immune system is a sophisticated network of organs and functions that has developed to defend against illness. The immune system is composed of both cellular and molecular components. These components' functions are separated into two categories: responsive reactions, which are tailored to certain pathogens, and nonspecific mechanisms, which are intrinsic to an organism. The study of the elements that comprise the innate and adaptive immune systems is known as fundamental or classical immunology.

The initial line of defense is **innate immunity**, which is non-specific. In other words, regardless of how distinct each possible infection may be, the reactions are all the same. Physical barriers (skin, saliva, etc.) and cells (macrophages, neutrophils, basophils, mast cells, etc.) are examples of innate immunity. These "ready to go" components shield an organism during the initial days of infection. Sometimes this is sufficient to eradicate the infection, but other times the first line of defense is overpowered and a second line of defense is activated.

The second line of defense is **adaptive immunity**, which entails storing memories of illnesses experienced in order to produce a more effective response tailored to the pathogen or foreign material. Antibodies, which are a component of adaptive immunity, often target foreign pathogens that are free to traverse the bloodstream. T cells are also engaged; they can either directly kill infected cells or aid in regulating the antibody response. T cells are specifically targeted at infections that have colonized cells.

Clinical immunology and immune dysfunction

Disease can arise from a disruption in the immune system's delicate balance, which is closely regulated. This field of study focuses on illnesses brought on by immune system malfunction. By changing the way the immune system functions or, in the case of vaccines, priming the immune system and increasing the immunological response to particular infections, a large portion of this work is important for the development of new therapies and treatments that can control or cure the condition.

The immune system's capacity to mount a suitable defense is compromised in **immunodeficiency** diseases. Because of this, these conditions are nearly invariably linked to serious infections that last, recur, and/or cause complications, which can make them extremely incapacitating and even deadly. There are two kinds of immunodeficiency disorders: primary immunodeficiencies are extremely uncommon, usually present from birth, and usually inherited. Common variable immunodeficiency (CVID) is one such instance. As is the case with AIDS after HIV infection, secondary immunodeficiencies can arise after an infection and typically manifest later in life.

When the immune system targets the body it is supposed to defend, autoimmune disorders result. Individuals with **autoimmune illnesses** are defective in their ability to discriminate between "self" and "non-self" or "foreign" molecules. Numerous laboratory assays for autoimmune disease detection have been made possible by the concepts of immunology. There are two types of autoimmune diseases: "primary" autoimmune diseases, such as type 1 diabetes, which can appear at birth or in early life, and "secondary" autoimmune diseases, which appear later in life for a variety of reasons. This category of autoimmunity is believed to include multiple sclerosis and rheumatoid arthritis. Additionally, autoimmune disorders can be widespread, like systemic lupus erythematosus (SLE), or localized, like Crohn's disease, which affects the GI tract.

Allergies are hypersensitivity illnesses that happen when the body's immune system damages its own tissues in response to harmless outside substances. Allergies can be caused by almost anything (an allergen), although they usually start after eating certain foods (like peanuts) or breathing in dust or pollen from the air. When an allergic reaction occurs, the body instantly creates chemicals to combat the allergen because it perceives it as harmful. Strong chemicals like histamine are released by immune system cells as a result, leading to inflammation and a host of allergy symptoms. The goal of immunology is to comprehend what occurs in the body during an allergic reaction and the causes of these reactions. Better techniques for identifying, preventing, and managing allergy disorders should result from this.

Asthma is a crippling and occasionally fatal condition that affects the airways. It usually happens when the immune system reacts to airborne particles and can cause patients' airways to thicken over time. It is a leading cause of disease and is especially common in kids. There may be an allergic component in certain cases, but the underlying cause is more complicated and unclear in others.

The ability of **cancer** cells to evade immune destruction is one of the characteristics that identify cancer, a disease characterized by aberrant and unchecked cell growth and proliferation. Since immune system evasion has been linked to cancer, researchers have resorted to immunotherapy, which involves modifying the immune system to combat cancer. Cancer immunotherapy has demonstrated remarkable potential as a new tool in our fight against the disease. It aims to activate the immune system's natural defenses against malignant tissue. The use of monoclonal antibodies—proteins that seek for and directly attach to a specific target protein known as an antigen—is another way that immunological knowledge is applied to combat cancer. One such example is Herceptin, a monoclonal antibody used to treat stomach and breast cancer. Additionally, several effective cancer vaccinations, including the HPV vaccine, have been created.

Transplant: Transferring organs, tissues, or cells from a donor to a recipient is known as a transplant. The immune system's perception of the transplanted organs as alien is the biggest obstacle to transplantation. Determining a diagnosis, suggesting a course of treatment, and creating novel approaches and medications to manage transplants and reduce the risk of rejection all depend on an understanding of the mechanics and clinical characteristics of rejection.

Vaccines: The purpose of vaccines is to teach the body how to identify and protect itself from diseases caused by dangerous pathogens including bacteria, viruses, and parasites. A sneak 'taste' of a particular pathogen is given by vaccines, which prompts the body's immune system to get ready for infection. A harmless component of the infectious pathogen found in vaccines triggers the immune system to create a defense, starting with the creation of antibodies. In addition to producing antibodies that are particular to the inciting substance, vaccine-responsive cells multiply to create "memory cells." These memory cells can quickly respond to the threat by generating enough antibody when they come into contact with the infectious pathogen again. Eventually, pathogens within the body are eliminated, preventing additional infection. Due to the effective use of vaccines, a number of infectious illnesses, such as smallpox, measles, mumps, rubella, diphtheria, tetanus, whooping cough, TB, and polio, are no longer a concern in Europe.

Immunology in veterinary medicine

A subfield of immunology devoted to enhancing animal health is called veterinary immunology. Similar to humans, animals can get diseases from either immune system malfunctions or germs attempting to infiltrate their bodies. The welfare of farm, domestic, and wild animals is frequently threatened by a wide variety of harmful germs, viruses, and parasites. Animal illnesses can have a broad impact on human industries like agriculture and food production. Furthermore, zoonosis is the word for the natural transmission of many animal infections to humans and vice versa across the species barrier. Malaria, Lyme disease, and swine and avian influenza are among the well-known illnesses that are spread from animals and insects to people. For this reason, it is crucial that these disorders are appropriately managed. These steps lessen any potentially disastrous societal and economic repercussions in addition to stopping any more transmission to humans and other animals.

Pathology

The study and diagnosis of disease are the main goals of the medical science field of pathology. In clinical pathology, surgically removed organs, tissues (biopsy samples), bodily fluids, and occasionally the entire body (autopsy) are examined. A body specimen's gross anatomical composition, cell appearance employing chemical and immunological signs, genetic research, and gene markers are some of the factors that may be taken into account. The great majority of cancer diagnoses are done by pathologists, who specialize in a variety of illnesses, including cancer. To identify if a tissue sample is malignant or non-cancerous (benign), its cellular pattern is examined under a microscope.

Examining the causes, mechanisms, and severity of disease is part of pathology, a related scientific study of disease processes. Particular illnesses of the individual organ systems are studied, along with cellular adaptation to injury, necrosis (death of live cells or tissues), inflammation, wound healing, and neoplasia (abnormal new development of cells). In order to improve diagnosis and treatment, our research labs are dedicated to comprehending the cellular anomalies in disease. Candidates in our Graduate Studies Program receive training in disease laboratory research.

The recent renaming of the Royal College-recognized subspecialty from Anatomical Pathology to Diagnostic & Molecular Pathology in 2024 marks a significant milestone in the field of pathology, which has evolved from a macroscopic/microscopic to a molecular level understanding of human disease and precision medicine. This change demonstrates how pathology has emerged as a major force in patient treatment and prognosis, moving from a primarily diagnostic field to the forefront of health science innovation.

Pathology in surgery

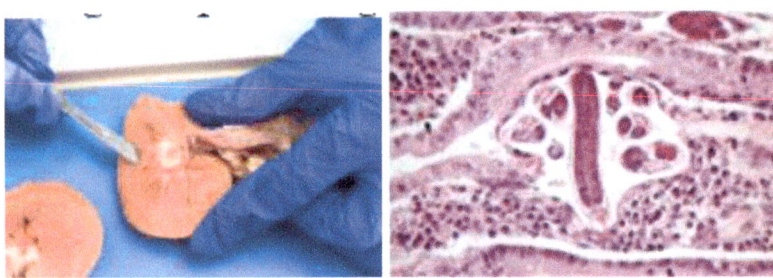

With a primary focus on analyzing tissues with the naked eye or under a microscope to provide a conclusive diagnosis of disease, surgical pathology is the most important and time-consuming area of pathology. Sources of surgically removed specimens include tiny skin biopsies, core biopsies used to diagnose cancer, and operating rooms where tumors are removed. Both macroscopic (gross) and microscopic (histologic) tissue examination are used in surgical pathology, where immunohistochemistry or other laboratory procedures are used to evaluate the molecular characteristics of tissue samples.

Either frozen sections or chemical fixation are used to prepare histological tissue sections for microscopic inspection. The technique of frozen section processing entails freezing the tissue to create thin, frozen specimen slices that are adhered to glass slides. Slides prepared by chemical fixation or frozen slice are either stained with chemicals or antibodies to reveal cellular components before the tissue is examined under a microscope.

A pathologist performs an **autopsy**, a highly specialized surgical technique that involves a comprehensive examination of a corpse to ascertain the cause and manner of death as well as to assess any potential injuries or diseases. Determining the cause of death, the individual's condition before to death, and whether any pre-death medical diagnosis and treatment were suitable are the main goals of an autopsy or post-mortem examination.

The study of cytopathology

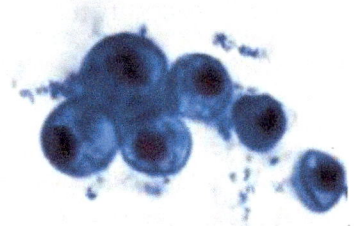

A subfield of pathology called cytopathology examines and diagnoses illnesses at the cellular level. It is typically used to assist diagnose cancer, but it can also be used to diagnose other inflammatory illnesses and some viral infections. Unlike histopathology, which examines entire tissues, cytopathology is typically applied to samples of free cells or tissue fragments that exfoliate spontaneously or are extracted from tissues by abrasion or small needle aspiration.

Molecular Pathology

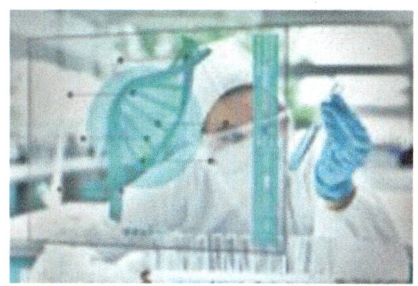

Over the past ten years, the relatively new field of molecular pathology has made impressive strides. It places a strong emphasis on using the analysis of chemicals found in organs, tissues, or physiological fluids to research and diagnose illness. Finding particular characteristic mutations enables clinicians to categorize an illness and select the best course of treatment. Many diseases, including cancer, are brought on by mutations or changes in an individual's genetic code. Therefore, by enabling us to forecast a patient's reaction to specific anti-cancer treatments based on their unique genetic composition, molecular analysis is setting the standard for customized medicine. Molecular pathology encompasses the creation of molecular and genetic methods for the diagnosis and categorization of human tumors as well as the creation and validation of predictive biomarkers for disease prognosis and an individual's vulnerability to developing specific cancers. Molecular tests' high sensitivity makes it possible to identify tiny tumors that would otherwise go undetected by other methods. This will probably lead to an earlier diagnosis, better patient care, and better survival rates.

Pathology Digital

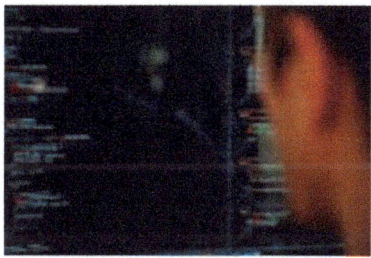

An emerging field of quantitative pathologic evaluation is called "digital pathology," which includes whole-slide scanners, new imaging technologies, slide digitization, and artificial intelligence (AI)-based analysis. Images and data can be stored and shared for remote education, research, consultation, and diagnostics, in addition to extracting information that is not visible to the human eye.

Pharmacology

The study of how medications affect a biologic system is known as pharmacology. It includes elements of biology and medicine as well as their interactions.

A drug is any chemical (natural, synthetic, or endogenous compounds) that affects a cell, tissue, or organ in the body. The term "drug" can refer to a wide range of substances.

Drugs' origins, properties, and effects—whether biologic, chemical, or therapeutic—on biological systems are all covered in pharmacology.

Pharmacy is not the same as pharmacology. The science of finding and characterizing drugs that affect the body is known as pharmacology.

Conversely, pharmacy describes medical services that apply pharmacological principles to enhance patient outcomes in a therapeutic context.

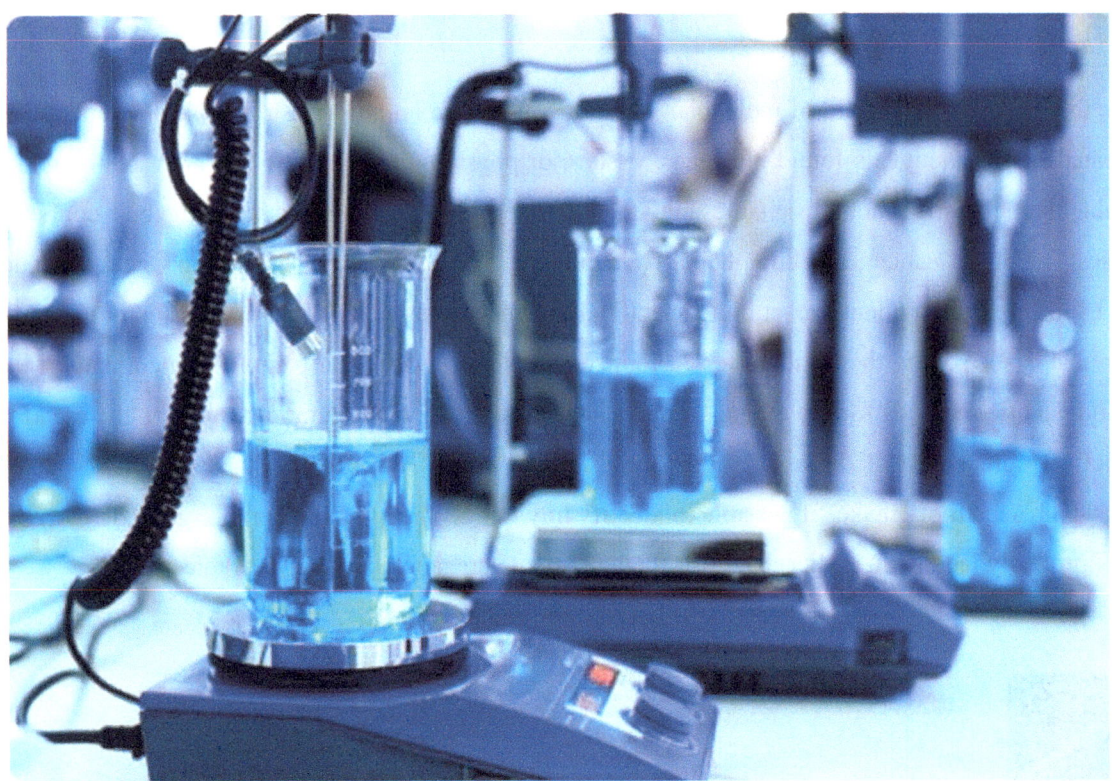

laboratory for medical pharmacology.

The past

Pharmaceuticals like morphine and quinine, which are typically derived from natural sources or plant extracts, have historically had their effects on the body poorly understood and described in generic terms without a thorough understanding of how they work.

William Withering (1741–1799) was one of the main pioneers of clinical pharmacology, a discipline that had roots in the Middle Ages. However, its advancement as a scientific field did not occur until the middle of the 19th century. The developments in biomedical science at the time were primarily to blame for this.

As a biological discipline, pharmacology developed further during the 19th and 20th centuries, and its findings were first used in therapeutic settings.

Pharmacologists today understand and control the pharmacological activity of drugs for medical reasons using a range of methods, such as chemistry, molecular biology, and genetics. Over the past century, this has contributed to significant advancements in the field of medicine.

It has led to a better comprehension of the ways in which drugs can be utilized to treat a range of illnesses and ailments.

Topics in Pharmacology

Numerous subjects are covered in the wide-ranging field of pharmacology. These consist of:

- The makeup of drugs
- Properties of drugs
- Drug production and illness
- The cellular and molecular processes by which drugs work
- Mechanisms of the body and organ systems
- Cellular communication, including signal transduction
- Molecular diagnostics
- Interactions between drugs
- The study of toxicology
- Chemical biology
- Medication
- Uses in medicine

Pharmaceutical kinetics and pharmacodynamics

The two main branches of pharmacology are pharmacodynamics and pharmacokinetics. The study of pharmacodynamics focuses on how a medicine may affect the body's biochemistry. Pharmacokinetics is more concerned with how the drug is absorbed, metabolized, distributed, and eliminated by the body.

Pharmacodynamics is the study of how drugs interact with the body's receptors and how these interactions can be advantageous for specific goals.

The study of pharmacokinetics examines the body's response to the introduction of pharmacological compounds into the body's systems. The four primary subjects of this are medication absorption, distribution throughout the body, metabolism into other compounds, and excretion from the body (also known as ADME).

Sub-disciplines

Pharmacology encompasses a wide range of sub-disciplines and specializations. These consist of:

- Cardiovascular pharmacology is the study of how medications affect the heart.
- therapeutic pharmacology: the use of drugs in therapeutic settings
- Dental pharmacology is the study of how medications are used to treat dental conditions.
- Environmental pharmacology: comprehending how genes, the environment, and medications interact
- Pharmacological impacts on the central and peripheral nervous systems are known as neuropharmacology.
- Pharmacoepidemiology: the study of how drugs affect sizable populations
- Pharmacogenetics: the connection between drug response and genetic variability
- Pharmacogenomics: the discovery and characterization of drugs using genetic technology
- The study of pharmaceutical composition, application, and development is known as pharmacognosy.

- Posology: the study of determining the appropriate dosage for medications
- Psychopharmacology: the alterations in behaviour linked to drugs or the application of drugs to alter behaviour
- The use of a system's biologic principles to adjust medications is known as systems pharmacology.
- The theory behind the impact of novel medications is known as theoretical pharmacology.
- Toxicology: the negative consequences of drugs

If a pharmacologist wants to delve deeper into a particular field of pharmacology, they can specialize in any one of these sub-disciplines.

The "National Statement on Ethical Conduct in Human Research" and its effects on behavioural science ethics

This book delves deeply into the ethics of behaviour change, providing answers to topics such as why ethics matter and how the "National Statement on Ethical Conduct in Human Research" relates to my work as a behaviour change practitioner.

Australia's ethical foundation for conducting research involving human subjects is known as the "National Statement on Ethical Conduct in Human Research." It could seem quite technical and unrelated to the tasks you conduct on a daily basis. However, ethics is broad and involves doing everything in a way that is ethically correct or appropriate.

Therefore, you, like everyone else, have a moral commitment to do good and refrain from harming others, even if your job is not categorized as "research." The ability of behavioural science to alter people's behaviour is another reason to think about the ethics of your job if it entails changing behaviour.

In 2023, the National Statement was modified by the Australian Government (NHMRC), primarily in the areas of governance and ethics review (Section 5) and risks and benefits of research involvement. For the former, risk is currently categorized for any "harmful" research activities on a continuum from low risk to high risk. This new classification calls for ethics review boards to give careful thought to high-risk cases, which include re-traumatization from research-related anxiety and even death.

However, at best, research activities conducted by behavioural scientists and practitioners may cause participants to experience annoyance. For example, in an effort to measure this behaviour, they would ask their participants to track how long they spend in the shower for a week. Additional instances include completing questionnaires or paying for travel expenses. The National Statement states that since these activities are no longer dangerous, they do not qualify as risk. However, practitioners, researchers, and ethics review boards should continue to balance these risks against the advantages of involvement in cases where minimal or low risk or damage is predictable.

Why is ethics important?

Ethics is important to behavioural science practitioners for a variety of reasons. Possibly the most important factor has to do with the ability we acquire to gather and consider "audience insights" while making decisions. In other words, we gather first-hand information on human behaviour and its causes in order to guide the design of interventions. The techniques used to gather this data are frequently comparable, if not the same as, those employed by researchers. These techniques include designing and disseminating surveys; interviewing people and posing questions; and seeing people in action to learn more about their behaviour. A variety of ethical norms, including autonomy and dignity, privacy and secrecy, beneficence (behaving in the best interests of others), and nonmaleficence (doing no harm), must be carefully considered when conducting such research operations.

In a broader sense, ethics also play a significant role in choosing the issues you will work on, the partners you will collaborate with, the behaviours you hope to change, and the methods you will use to do it. Different personal ideals, professional standards and values, organizational policies, and social or cultural conventions can all serve as our compass. There will already be well-established ethical standards, regulations, and infrastructure in place in some, but not all, fields of professional research and practice. Although it has less to say about whether or not we conduct behaviour change interventions—in fact, there is currently no regulatory agency for this—the National Statement is nonetheless a helpful tool to assist strong ethical decisions in research.

Therefore, we surveyed the participants in our behaviour modification course in early 2022 and asked them these two questions. The goal was to comprehend the various viewpoints that practitioners have while considering the ethics of behaviour modification. After analyzing 52 de-identified replies, we discovered the following overall results:

1. In response to the question, "Do you have the authority to alter citizens' behaviour? 90% of respondents agreed that humans should have the ability to alter their behaviour, but only under specific ethical guidelines. The majority of respondents (77%) specifically mentioned the desire to "do good" in their response, indicating that they only believed they had the authority to alter their behaviour if doing so would benefit the individual or society as a whole.
2. In response to the question, "Is it appropriate to employ any kind of tool to modify behaviour as long as it benefits the individual or society? Approximately equal proportions of replies touched on the ideals of respect, justice, and openness as conditions in the use of any instrument, with the majority (96%) disagreeing that any tool was suitable.

What can I do, then, to improve my ethical mindset in my behaviour modification efforts?

It is crucial to thoroughly assess the ethical implications of your work and implement as many of the principles as possible while planning and designing your behaviour change interventions, even though there may not be a simple or prescriptive solution to every particular ethical problem.

Using a variety of ethical frameworks and behavioural science norms, we have developed a set of questions that all practitioners should consider before starting any behaviour modification initiative:

1. Is behavioural science a suitable strategy for reaching your objective? Do you need someone to approach your problem or challenge in a new way? Is there another method to fix your problem?
2. Will your target audience's lives be better as a result of your behaviour change intervention? Will the individuals involved in your campaign ultimately gain more if you consider the risks and rewards of participating?
3. Does your behaviour change intervention have clear and open goals, aims, and purposes? Respect is one of the core ethical criteria that can be met when you give the target audience the information they require to determine whether or not to participate in your campaign. Being open and honest also helps you stay aware of dishonest, manipulative, or cryptic activities.

4. Does your behaviour modification program honour people's autonomy and sense of dignity? Respect also entails appreciating human agency and judgment. Respect and fairness can be shown by abstaining from offensive or discriminating actions and practices.
5. 5. Is fairness maintained by your behavioural intervention? We frequently give preferential treatment to our target audiences in an attempt to assist them, thus causing disadvantages and inequality among other groups. Think about how much your intervention ignores one group and concentrates too much on another. Is this fair?
6. Lastly, do you have enough procedures and plans in place for evaluation and to spot any unfavourable effects of your behaviour modification intervention? Even while we try our best to make well-informed judgments in our behaviour change efforts and to embrace the values of beneficence, justice, respect, and dignity, can we be certain that we are succeeding if we are not monitoring?

Therefore, it is only professional to carry out your task with integrity if it entails collaborating with people, gathering information from them, or attempting to influence their behaviour. We can all contribute to making the world a better, more equitable place by taking the time to review the ethical concepts that are pertinent to your line of work, making sure that different viewpoints are included at crucial stages of decision-making, and sense-checking research plans or intervention designs.

Section 2

Systems-Based Approach

What to know about the cardiovascular system

The heart, blood arteries, and blood make up the cardiovascular system. Its main job is to provide oxygen-rich blood and nutrients to every area of the body while returning deoxygenated blood to the lungs.

Serious health issues may arise from abnormalities or damage to any or all of the cardiovascular system's components. Heart attacks, strokes, high blood pressure, and coronary artery disease are common disorders that can impact the cardiovascular system.

The cardiovascular system, including its parts and their roles, is examined in this book. We also include a few common ailments of the cardiovascular system and the treatments for them.

The cardiovascular system's components

The system in charge of supplying blood to the various body parts is the cardiovascular system. It is composed of the following tissues and organs:

- The heart: The body's muscular pump that circulates blood.
- A closed network of blood vessels, comprising:
  - Arteries: Blood vessels that leave the heart.
  - The vessels that return blood to the heart are called veins.
  - Capillaries: Small blood vessels that emerge from arteries to supply blood to every bodily tissue.

The body has two blood circulation systems. The systemic circulatory system is the first. This is the primary blood circulation system that carries blood to all of the body's organs, tissues, and cells.

The pulmonary circulation system comes in second. Blood is transported from the heart to the lungs by this circulatory system. It is the point at which carbon dioxide exits the blood and oxygen enters.

The heart's structure

Two upper chambers known as "atria" and two bottom chambers known as "ventricles" make up the heart's four independent chambers. The atria and ventricles are divided by a wall known as the "septum." The flow of blood between the various chambers is managed via valves.

The flow of blood via the heart is as follows:

1. Via the inferior and superior vena cava veins, blood deficient in oxygen leaves the body and reaches the right atrium, or upper right chamber.
2. After passing through the tricuspid valve, blood reaches the lower right chamber of the right ventricle.
3. Through the pulmonary valve and the major pulmonary artery, the right ventricle pumps blood out of the heart.

4. After that, the blood enters the lungs via the left and right pulmonary arteries. In this case, breathing takes carbon dioxide out of the blood and brings oxygen into it. The blood is now rich in oxygen as a result.
5. Four pulmonary veins carry the blood back to the heart and into the left atrium, or upper left chamber.
6. Blood enters the left ventricle (lower left chamber) after passing through the mitral valve.
7. The aortic valve allows the left ventricle to pump blood into the "aorta," a major artery that supplies blood to the rest of the body.

The significance of the heart

Every tissue in the body receives blood from the heart via closed arteries. All of the body's cells subsequently receive nutrition and oxygen from the blood itself. The tissues and cells would not be able to perform at their best without blood, and they would start to malfunction and eventually perish.

What is the cardiac cycle?

There are two stages in the cardiac cycle.

The ventricles fill with blood during the first phase, known as diastole. It starts with the closure of the aortic or pulmonary valve and finishes with the closure of the mitral or tricuspid valve. Blood vessels return blood to the heart during diastole so that the ventricles can contract again.

Systole is the second stage, during which the ventricles contract and release blood. It starts with the closure of the tricuspid or mitral valve and finishes with the closure of the aortic or pulmonary valve. Blood is forced from the ventricles to the vessels when the pressure inside the ventricles exceeds the pressure inside nearby blood vessels.

Typical cardiovascular disorders

Severe cardiovascular conditions have the potential to be fatal. People may be better able to obtain prompt and appropriate medical counsel if they are aware of the disorders that can impact the cardiovascular system.

Below are summaries of a few prevalent cardiovascular conditions.

A heart attack

When there is insufficient blood flow to a portion of the heart muscle, a heart attack occurs. A blockage, a rupture in an artery around the heart, or the heart needing more oxygen than is available can all cause this.

Heart attack symptoms include:

- Pain or discomfort in the chest
- Experiencing dizziness
- Back, neck, or jaw pain or discomfort
- Soreness or pain in one or both shoulders or arms
- Breathing difficulties

The following are three major heart attack risk factors:

- elevated cholesterol in the blood
- elevated blood pressure
- Smoking

Heart attack survivors can reduce their risk of developing cardiovascular issues in the future by doing the following:

- Consistent physical exercise
- Getting to or staying at a modest weight
- Adhering to a diet that promotes heart health
- Giving up smoking
- going through cardiac rehabilitation

A stroke

A stroke is a medical disease where a portion of the brain loses its blood flow. The death of brain cells is brought on by this lack of blood flow.

Two kinds of stroke exist. A blood clot obstructing blood flow to the brain causes an ischemic stroke. A hemorrhage in or around the brain causes a hemorrhagic stroke.

The following are some important stroke risk factors:

- elevated blood pressure
- Diabetes
- Heart conditions
- Smoking
- A history of stroke in one's family or personally
- advanced age
- Having African American ancestry

The following are examples of sudden onset stroke symptoms:

- One-sided facial, arm, or leg weakness or numbness
- Issues with one or both eyes' vision
- Having trouble understanding or speaking
- Perplexity
- lightheadedness, unsteadiness, or trouble walking
- A rather bad headache

The type of stroke will determine the course of treatment. In order to assist break up the blood clot and restore blood flow to the brain, a person who has an ischemic stroke may be prescribed medicine. Surgery may be necessary to repair the bleeding blood vessel in a person who has a hemorrhagic stroke.

Treatments for stroke follow-up could include:

- Anticoagulant or antiplatelet drugs to help stop new blood clots from forming
- Blood pressure-lowering drugs
- drugs known as statins that lower blood cholesterol levels
- Physical treatment
- therapy for rehabilitation
- Speech therapy

Heart failure

When the heart cannot pump enough blood to meet the body's needs, heart failure results.

Among the signs of cardiac failure are:

- Constant wheezing or coughing
- Breathing difficulties
- Show intolerance
- A higher heart rate
- queasy
- A lack of hunger
- enlargement
- Weary
- Perplexity

Heart failure risk factors include:

- elevated blood pressure
- The condition of coronary arteries
- A history of one of the conditions listed below:
  - A heart attack
  - Diabetes
  - Apnea in sleep
  - A congenital cardiac condition

Heart failure has no known remedy. However, therapies can help to reduce symptoms and limit the disease's course. Among the examples are:

- Modifications to one's diet and level of exercise
- Instruments and surgical techniques
- Drugs used to control cholesterol or blood pressure
- Diuretics to lessen edema, or swelling

Arrhythmia

An irregular heartbeat is called an arrhythmia. It could show up as an abnormally fast or sluggish heartbeat or as a characteristic pattern. Symptoms could consist of:

- Is your heartbeat quick or slow?
- Skipping beats
- dizziness
- lightheadedness
- fainting
- Pain in the chest
- Breathing difficulties
- Sweating

Among the arrhythmia risk factors are:

- Heart conditions
- a birth defect of the heart
- elevated blood pressure
- elevated cholesterol
- advanced age
- The use of alcohol
- Sleep apnea left untreated

A pacemaker is a device that doctors may implant to restore a normal heart beat in cases of serious arrhythmias.

The impact of aging on the cardiovascular system

A person's heart starts to function less efficiently as they become older. For instance, while the resting heart rate is constant, it is unable to beat as quickly when exercising. As the heart ages, arrhythmias may also occur.

Increasing stiffness in the cardiac muscle and major arteries is another prevalent aging issue. High blood pressure brought on by this stiffness raises the risk of heart attacks, strokes, and heart failure. Congestive heart failure can also result from cardiac stiffness.

In brief

The heart, veins, arteries, and capillaries make up the cardiovascular system. The systemic and pulmonary circulatory systems are the two circulatory systems composed of these elements. Systole, or relaxation, and diastole, or contraction, are the two stages of the cardiac cycle.

Heart attack, stroke, heart failure, and arrhythmia are a few disorders that can impact the heart.

The heart's efficiency declines with age, particularly when the body is subjected to intense physical exercise. Additionally, as people age, their arteries are more likely to stiffen, raising the risk of high blood pressure and related cardiovascular problems.

Respiratory System

Your lungs, airways (trachea, bronchi, and bronchioles), diaphragm, voice box, throat, nose, and mouth comprise your respiratory system. Inhaling oxygen and exhaling carbon dioxide are its primary functions. Along with enabling speech and scent, it also helps shield you from dangerous particles and pathogens.

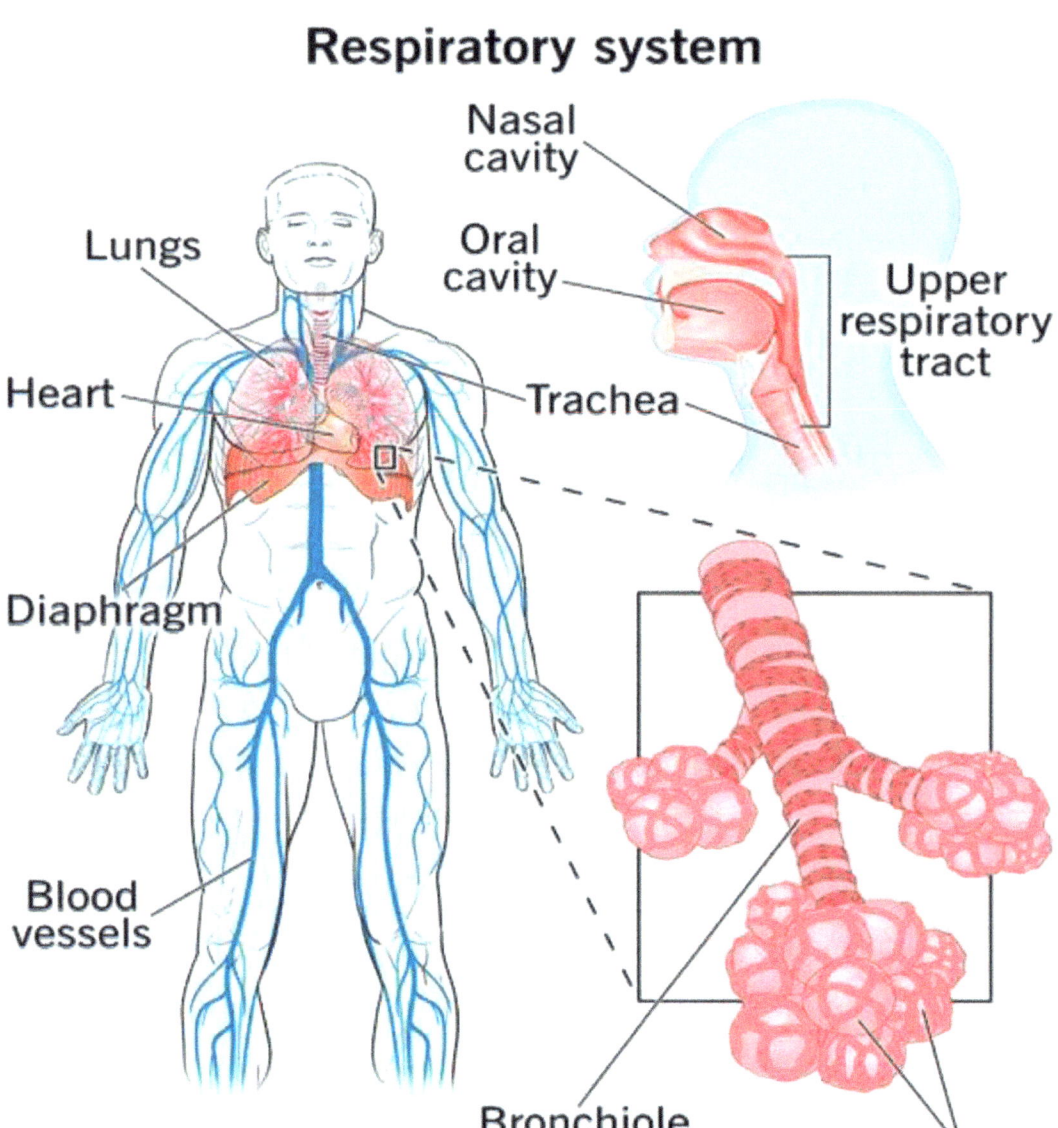

The lungs, airways, pharynx, larynx, nose, and mouth are the parts of your respiratory system that take in oxygen and expel carbon dioxide.

What is the respiratory system?

The organs and tissues in your body that enable breathing are called your respiratory system. It consists of the tube-like structures (airways) that connect your mouth, nose, and lungs. Your respiratory system is supported by blood vessels and muscles, and it is shielded by your ribs. Together, these components allow your body to absorb oxygen during inhalation and expel carbon dioxide during exhalation.

Operation

What is your respiratory system's primary purpose?

Your respiratory system's primary job is to remove carbon dioxide, a waste product, and draw in oxygen for your body's cells. This is accomplished by breathing in and out as well as by gas exchange between the blood arteries that run close by and the tiny air sacs in your lungs, known as alveoli. Additionally, your respiratory system:

- **Provides moisture and warmth to the air you breathe.** The air is warmed by your respiratory system to the temperature of your body. It hydrates the air to the proper humidity level for your body.
- **Guards your body against airborne contaminants.** Your respiratory system has components that can either keep dangerous bacteria and irritants out or force them out if they do get inside.
- **Permits you to speak.** Your voice chords vibrate in the air, producing sounds.
- **Aids in your ability to smell.** Your olfactory nerve, which communicates with your brain about odors, is traversed by the molecules in air when you breathe it in.
- **Regulates your body's acidity level.** Your blood becomes acidic when you have too much carbon dioxide in it. Your respiratory system contributes to the preservation of your body's acid-base equilibrium by eliminating carbon dioxide.

The anatomy

Which components make up the respiratory system?

Your lungs are the primary respiratory system organs. To help you breathe, however, your respiratory system is made up of numerous components. Your respiratory system is composed of the following parts:

- The nasal cavity and nose.
- The oral cavity and mouth.
- The sinuses.
- The throat (pharynx).
- The larynx, or voice box.
- The windpipe, or trachea.
- Large airways, or bronchi.
- The lungs.
- The diaphragm.

What is the upper respiratory tract like for you?

Air enters your body through your upper respiratory tract, which also assists in directing it toward your lungs. It gives the air you breathe more moisture. You draw air into your body through your mouth and nose, which is where your respiratory tract begins. Your larynx, sinuses (hollow spots on your forehead and cheeks), and nasal cavity are other components of your upper respiratory tract.

Which lower respiratory tract do you have?

The trachea, bronchi, and lungs make up the lower respiratory tract. the tracheobronchial (pronounced "tray-key-oh-BRON-key-uhl") tree is a network of progressively smaller tubes that carry air from the upper respiratory tract to tiny air sacs in your lungs (alveoli). It is composed of your trachea, bronchi, and bronchioles (small airways). (It resembles an upside-down tree in appearance.)

What is the function of your respiratory system?

For your cells to produce energy, oxygen is necessary. Carbon dioxide is a waste product released during energy production, and if it accumulates too much, it can be harmful to your health. Your respiratory system's primary function is gas exchange, which involves moving carbon dioxide out of your lungs and bringing oxygen into them. It accomplishes this by collaborating closely with your circulatory system, which includes your heart, blood, and blood vessels.

Every time you breathe in, imagine the oxygen in the air as passengers flying into your lungs from millions of planes. As your diaphragm descends, your chest expands, drawing air—along with its little oxygen cargo—into your lungs. Like airport runways, the air passes via your mouth or nose and down your trachea, bronchi, and bronchioles. The travelers then reach your alveoli, the airport gates.

There, the oxygen enters tiny blood vessels called capillaries through the membranes encircling your lungs. Consider it similar to the oxygen passengers being picked up at the airport by a cab. Ultimately, the cab makes its way to your tissues, where it drops off oxygen to power your cells.

How carbon dioxide is expelled from your respiratory system

Carbon dioxide is produced by cells when they consume energy. Carbon dioxide molecules enter your tissues when oxygen exits the taxi. They then make their way to the airport gates in your lungs via your bloodstream. When your diaphragm shifts back upward, your chest cavity shrinks and you force the air out the direction it came in, sending them flying out of your lungs.

Additional roles

Your respiratory system also shields your body from potentially dangerous particles and dry air when you breathe in and out. Your sinuses aid in controlling the air's temperature and humidity as you breathe in.

Tiny hairs called cilia filter away dust, bacteria, and other irritants as air passes through your nostrils and down your airways, preventing them from entering your lungs. Your respiratory system traps bacteria and irritants in mucus when they do manage to get inside. When you cough or sneeze, the cilia in your airways then move in a wave-like pattern to force the mucus out of your body.

Disorders and Conditions

Which illnesses have an impact on your respiratory system?

The tissues and organs that comprise your respiratory system might be impacted by a variety of illnesses. Some of these disorders can be brought on by irritants and microorganisms that you breathe in from the air, such as bacteria, viruses, and fungi that cause illnesses. Others are brought on by harm or inherited illnesses.

Your respiratory system may be impacted by the following conditions:

- **Rhinitis due to allergies.** Your nasal passageways and airways may be impacted by allergic reactions to dust, pet dander, tree pollen, and other allergens.
- **Prolonged respiratory disorders.** These include cystic fibrosis, asthma, and chronic obstructive pulmonary disease (COPD).
- **Infections of the upper and lower respiratory tract.** Colds and the flu (influenza) are frequent respiratory diseases.
- **Inflammation.** A respiratory infection may cause swelling in your sinuses (sinusitis), alveoli (pneumonia), or big airways (bronchitis).
- **ILD, or interstitial lung disease.** Your lungs may be permanently scarred by pulmonary fibrosis and other ILDs.
- **Obstacles.** This can be a malignant tumor, a benign growth, or an alien item.
- **Unbalances in acid-base.** Exhaling too much or too little carbon dioxide can cause respiratory alkalosis and acidosis, which alter the blood's acid-base balance.
- **Your blood or tissues contain either too much carbon dioxide or too little oxygen.** Hypoxemia, hypoxia, and hypercapnia can all indicate a respiratory system problem, even though they may appear to be blood disorders.

What symptoms may an illness affecting your respiratory system present with?

Your respiratory system may be affected by conditions that lead to:

- Dyspnea, or shortness of breath.
- A stuffy or runny nose.
- Cyanosis, or blue skin, lips, or nails.

Which tests are used by medical professionals to identify respiratory disorders?

To assess the condition of your respiratory system, medical professionals employ a variety of tests and procedures. These could include the following, depending on your symptoms:

- Pulse ox, or pulse oximetry. This is a straightforward, everyday test that measures your blood oxygen level using a device on your finger.
- Tests of pulmonary function.
- X-rays of the chest.
- Blood gas in the arteries.

Which therapies are frequently used to treat respiratory disorders?

The kind and severity of your respiratory ailment will determine the therapies you receive. Among the possible treatments are:

- Inhaled bronchodilators or corticosteroids. You may use an inhaler on a regular basis if you have asthma, COPD, or other disorders that cause your airways to constrict.
- Drugs for infections that are antiviral, antibiotic, or antifungal.
- Antihistamines.
- The modifiers of leukotriene.
- Rehabilitation for the lungs.
- Tumor or other obstruction surgery.
- A lung transplant.

Take care

How can I maintain the health of my respiratory system?

To maintain the health of your respiratory system:

- Don't vape or smoke. Smoking either causes or exacerbates a number of lung and airway conditions. Many of the chemicals found in cigarettes are also found in vaping liquids.
- Steer clear of contaminants that can harm your respiratory system. This includes chemicals, radon (a radioactive gas that can cause cancer), and secondhand smoke. If your profession or hobbies expose you to dust, fumes, or other pollutants, wear a mask.
- Drink plenty of water. The mucus in your lungs stays thin and is simpler to expel when you drink a lot of water.
- Engage in regular exercise. Exercise facilitates easy breathing and maintains the strength of your lungs' muscles.
- Avoid becoming sick. Getting immunized against respiratory diseases and washing your hands frequently will help keep you healthy.

When should I contact a medical professional?

If you experience shortness of breath, a persistent or worsening cough, or other signs of a respiratory disease, get in touch with your healthcare professional. See your provider for routine examinations. Respiratory problems can be kept from getting worse with early detection.

A message

Inhale. Exhale. You can center and relax by breathing. In addition to helping you taste and smell, it even lets you sing along to your favorite tune. Above all, your respiratory system removes carbon dioxide from your body to prevent it from building up and brings in oxygen to power your cells. If there is a problem with your respiratory system, you may cough, wheeze, or experience shortness of breath. Any symptoms that seem troubling should be discussed with your healthcare physician. They can ease your breathing.

Gastrointestinal Tract

Definition of the Gastrointestinal Tract

The portion of an organ system in humans and other animals that takes in food, breaks it down, absorbs nutrients, and then excretes it as feces is called the gastrointestinal tract.

Diagram of the Gastrointestinal Tract

The oral cavity, oesophagus, stomach, intestines, and anus are among the several tract components depicted in the gastrointestinal diagram below.

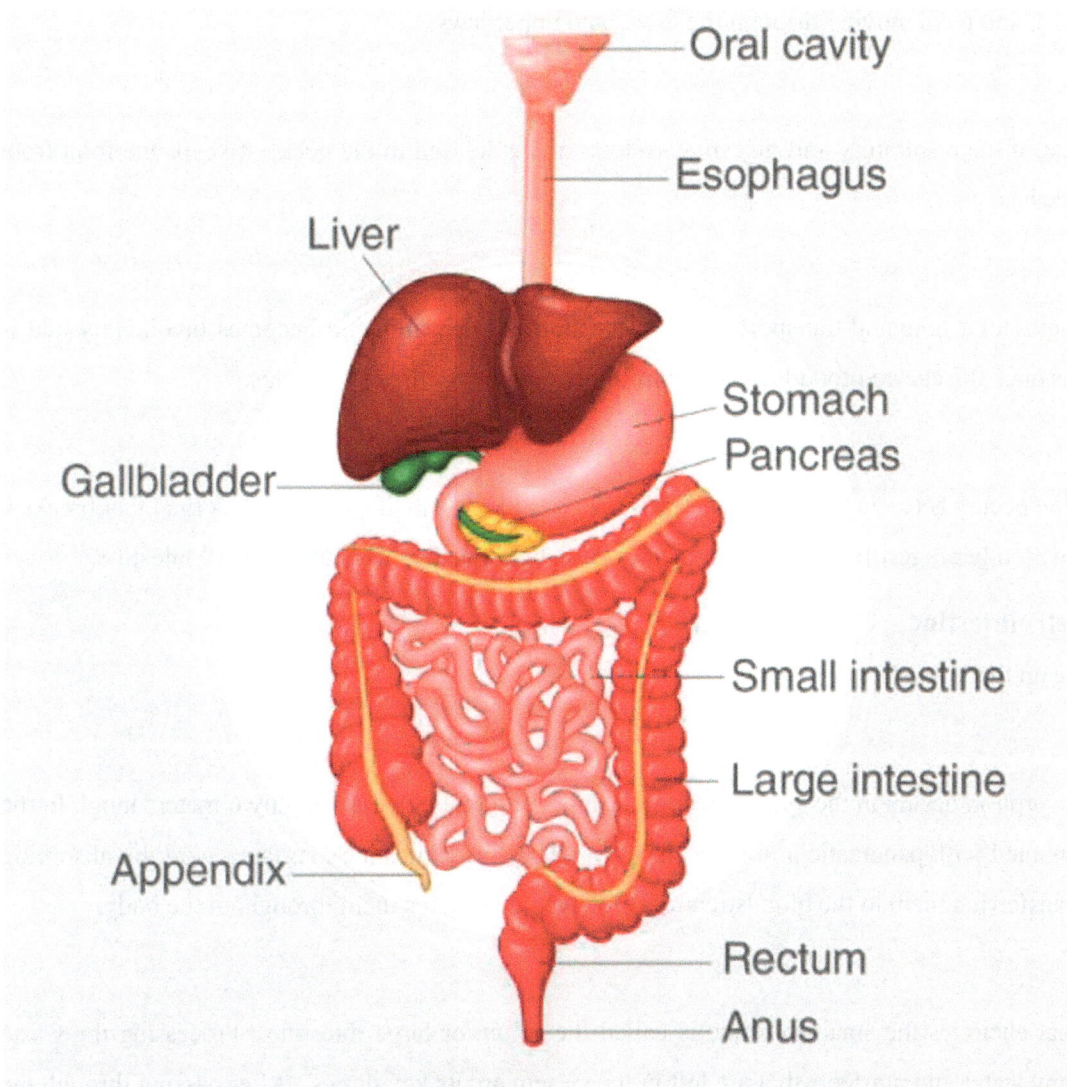

The anatomy of the gastrointestinal tract

In humans, the oesophagus, stomach, small and large intestines, and mouth make up the gastrointestinal system. The length of the GI tract is approximately 9 meters.

There are numerous supporting organs, including the liver, which aids in food digestion by secreting enzymes.

There are two parts to the human gastrointestinal tract, which are as follows:
- The upper gastrointestinal tract
- A smaller gastrointestinal tract

Gastrointestinal Tract Upper

The following organs make up the upper GI:

The mouth

Along with the soft palate, floor of the mouth, and bottom of the tongue, it also consists of the teeth, tongue, and buccal mucous membranes, which house the ends of the salivary glands. Food is continuously chewed in the mouth by the muscles of the tongue, cheeks, and teeth moving through the lower and upper jaws.

The Pharynx

The pharynx is a component of the respiratory and digestive systems and is housed in the neck. It keeps the food from getting into the lungs and trachea.

The oesophagus

an organ that resembles a muscular tube and transports food to the stomach. Swallowing becomes involuntary and is regulated by the oesophagus once the chewed food has passed from the mouth into the oesophagus.

The stomach

The majority of the digestion occurs here. Food is briefly stored in the stomach, a J-shaped bag-like organ that breaks it down, churns and mixes it with other digesting fluids and enzymes, and then transfers it on to the small intestine.

Tract of the Lower Gastrointestine

The following organs make up the lower GI:

The small intestine

The majority of nutrient absorption occurs in the small intestine, a thin, coiled tube that is roughly 6 meters long. In the small intestine, food is combined with pancreatic and liver enzymes. The small intestine's surfaces work by absorbing nutrients from meals and transferring them to the bloodstream, which then distributes them throughout the body.

Big Intestine

The thick tubular organ that encircles the small intestine is called the colon, or large intestine. Processing the waste materials and reabsorbing any water and nutrients that are left in the system are its key duties. After passing through the rectum, the leftover waste is expelled from the body as stool.

An infection of the gastrointestinal tract

Viruses, bacteria, and parasites that cause gastroenteritis and gastrointestinal tract inflammation can all cause intestinal infections. These have the potential to infect the small intestine as well as the stomach.

Microorganisms such as Staphylococcus aureus, E. coli, campylobacter, and adenovirus can cause these infections.

Diseases of the Gastrointestinal Tract

Among the illnesses of the gastrointestinal tract are:

Constipation

Infrequent or insufficient bowel movements are referred to as constipation. This is brought on by insufficient intake of water and dietary fiber.

Syndrome of Irritable Bowels

The colon muscle contracts more frequently in this situation than in healthy individuals. It results in diarrhea, cramping and pain in the abdomen, bloating, etc.

Cancer of the colon

Older adults are susceptible to colon cancer, which starts in the large intestine. It starts out as little, non-cancerous clusters. Over time, these clusters develop into cancer. Radiation therapy, chemotherapy, and surgery are available treatments.

Haemorrhoids

These are enlarged blood vessels that border the anus's orifice. They are brought on by too much pressure from the bowel's difficult motility.

Anatomy of the Urinary System

What is the function of the urinary system?

Urine is produced as a waste product after blood is filtered by the urinary system. The kidneys, renal pelvis, ureters, bladder, and urethra are the organs that make up the urinary system.

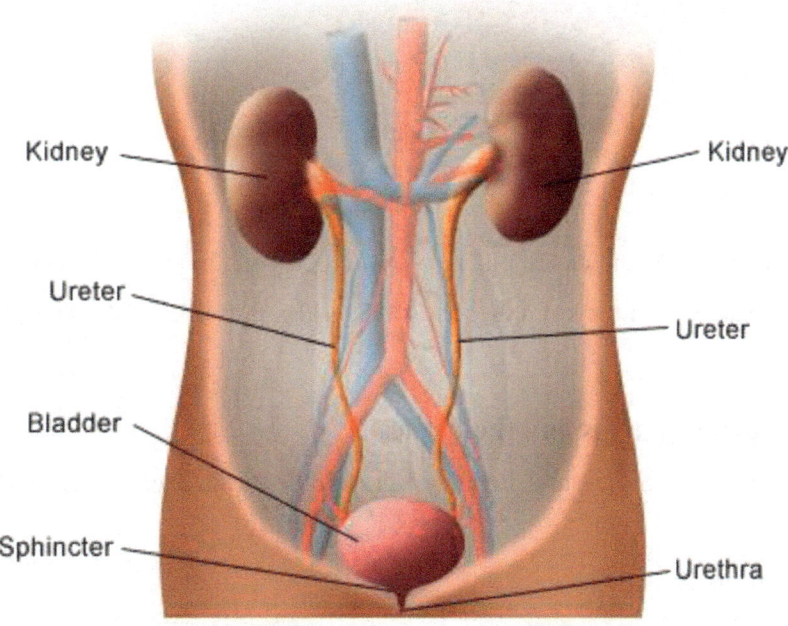

Food provides the body with nutrients, which it then transforms into energy. Waste products remain in the blood and in the bowel after the body has absorbed the necessary meal components.

The renal and urine systems assist the body in maintaining the proper balance of substances like potassium and sodium as well as water and in getting rid of liquid waste called urea. When the body breaks down protein-rich foods including meat, poultry, and some vegetables, urea is created. The bloodstream carries urea to the kidneys, where it is eliminated as urine together with water and other waste products.

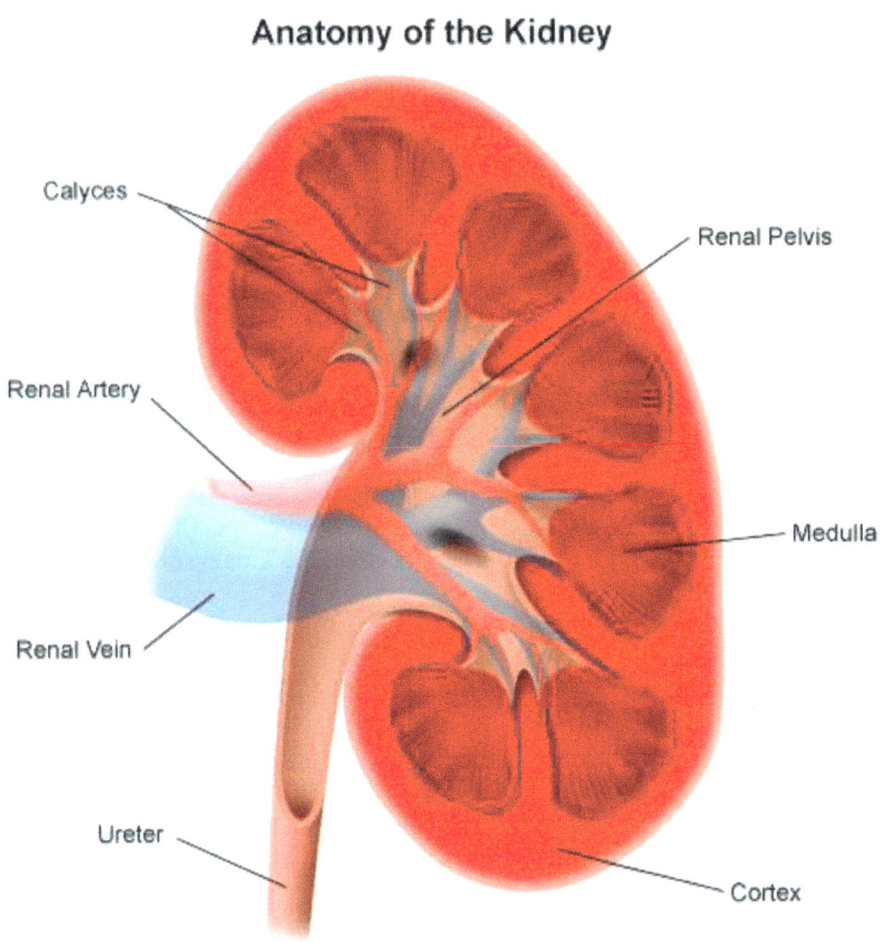

The production of erythropoietin, which regulates the development of red blood cells in the bone marrow, and blood pressure management are two further crucial roles of the kidneys. The kidneys also preserve fluids and control the acid-base balance.

The components of the kidney and urine systems and their roles
- Two kidneys. These two purplish-brown organs are situated in the middle of the back, beneath the ribs. Their role is to:
    o Eliminate medications and trash from the body.
    o Maintain the body's fluid balance
    o Issue hormones to control blood pressure.

o   Regulate the synthesis of red blood cells

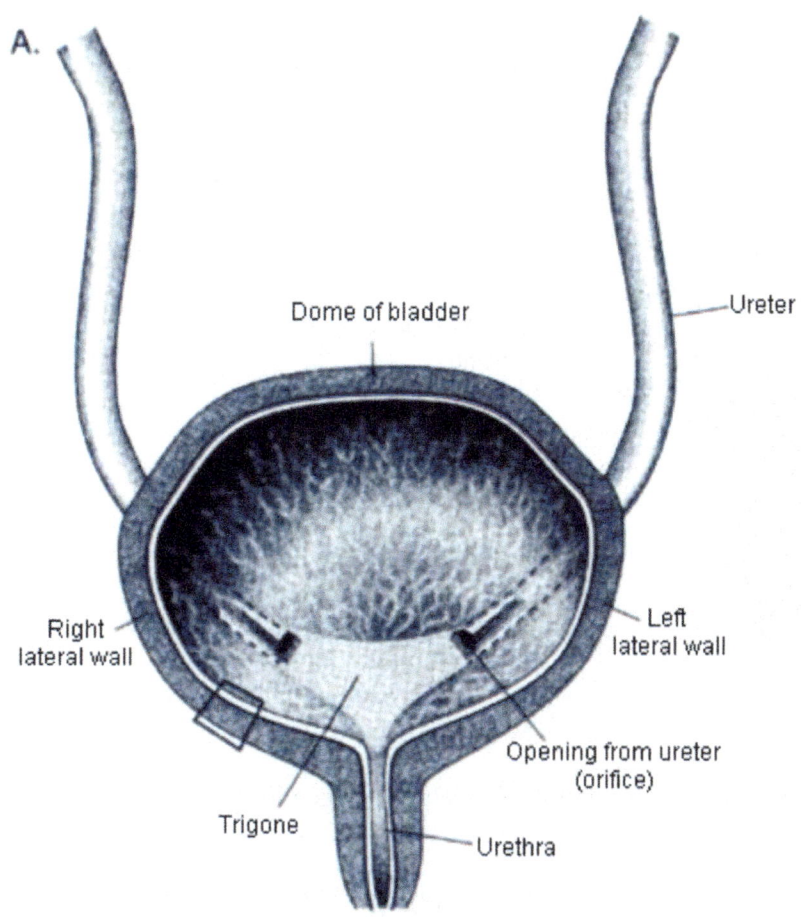

Nephrons are microscopic filtration units that the kidneys use to eliminate urea from the blood. Each nephron is made up of a renal tubule, which is a tiny tube, and a glomerulus, which is a ball made of tiny blood capillaries. As urine travels through the kidney's nephrons and renal tubules, it is composed of urea, water, and other waste materials.

- **Two ureters.** Urine is transported from the kidneys to the bladder via these slender tubes. Urine is forced downward and away from the kidneys by the constant tightening and relaxing of muscles in the ureter walls. A kidney infection may occur if the urine backs up or remains still. The ureters release tiny volumes of urine into the bladder every ten to fifteen seconds.
- **A bladder.** The lower abdomen contains this hollow, triangle-shaped organ. Ligaments that are connected to the pelvic bones and other organs hold it in place. The walls of the bladder compress and flatten to release pee through the urethra after relaxing and expanding to hold urine. Up to two cups of pee can be stored in the normal, healthy adult bladder for two to five hours.

When the bladder is examined, certain "landmarks" are utilized to indicate where any abnormalities may be found. They are:

o   Trigone: a triangle-shaped area close to where the bladder and urethra meet
o   The lateral walls on either side of the trigone are the right and left walls.

- o Back wall: posterior wall
- o Dome: the bladder's roof

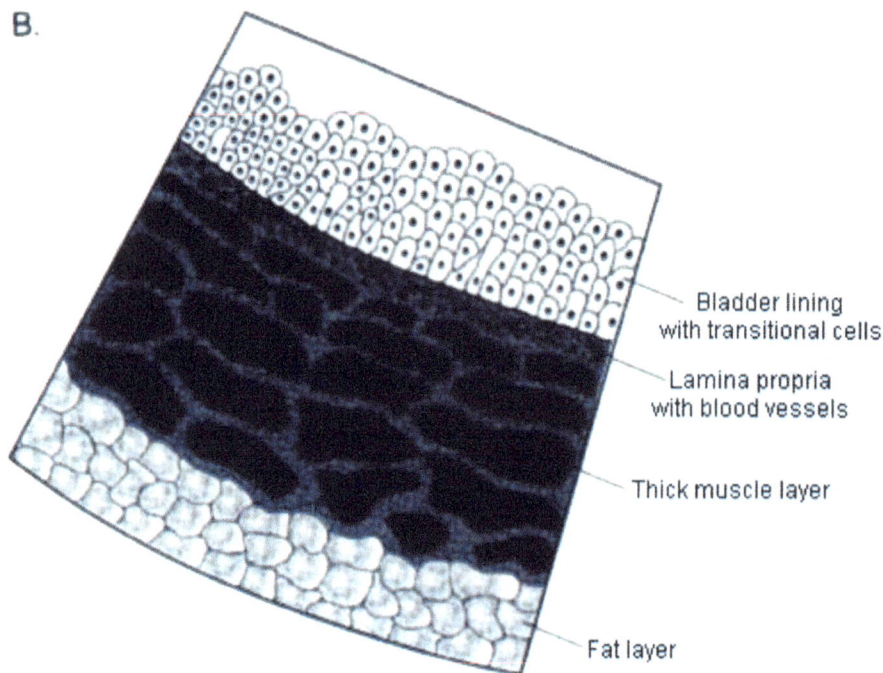

- **Two muscles called sphincters.** By tightly shutting around the bladder's entrance like a rubber band, these circular muscles assist prevent pee leaks.
- **The bladder nerves.** A person's nerves notify them when it's time to empty their bladder, or urinate.
- **The urethra.** Urine can exit the body through this tube. Urine is forced out of the bladder by the brain telling the muscles in the bladder to contract. Simultaneously, the brain instructs the sphincter muscles to relax, allowing urine to pass through the urethra from the bladder. Normal urination happens when all the signals appear in the right order.

Urine-related facts

- Clear yellow or pale straw is the color of normal, healthy pee.
- Urine that is darker yellow or honey in color indicates that you need more water.
- Severe dehydration or a liver issue may be indicated by a deeper, brownish hue.
- Urine that is crimson or pink could indicate blood in it.

The Endocrine System

Does the Endocrine System Exist?

Hormone-producing glands make up the endocrine system. The body uses hormones as chemical messengers. From one set of cells to another, they transport data and commands.

Nearly every cell, organ, and bodily function is influenced by the endocrine system, which is pronounced EN-duh-krin.

The Endocrine System: What Does It Do?

- Hormones are released into the bloodstream by endocrine glands. As a result, the hormones might reach cells in different areas of the body.
- The endocrine hormones regulate mood, growth and development, metabolism, reproduction, and the function of our organs.
- The amount of each hormone released is controlled by the endocrine system. This may rely on the blood's levels of other chemicals, such as calcium, or on the hormones that are already present. Stress, infections, and alterations in the fluid and mineral balance of the blood are just a few of the numerous factors that can impact hormone levels.

Any hormone in excess or insufficient amounts might be detrimental to the body. Many of these issues can be resolved with medication.

Which components make up the endocrine system?

The main glands that comprise the endocrine system are the following, while many other regions of the body also produce hormones:

- The hypothalamus
- Pituitary
- thyroid
- The parathyroids
- The adrenal glands
- The spinal body
- The ovaries

The testes

The pancreas is a component of both the digestive and endocrine systems. This is because it produces and secretes enzymes into the digestive system as well as hormones into the bloodstream.

Hypothalamus: The lower central region of the brain contains the hypothalamus, which is pronounced hi-po-THAL-uh-mus. It connects the nervous and endocrine systems. The hypothalamus's nerve cells produce substances that regulate the pituitary gland's hormone output. The pituitary receives information from the hypothalamus that the brain has sensed, including ambient temperature, light exposure, and emotions. The pituitary's production and release of hormones are influenced by this information.

Pituitary: The pituitary gland, which is about the size of a pea, is located near the base of the brain. Despite its little size, the pituitary is frequently referred to as the "master gland." Numerous other endocrine glands are regulated by the hormones it produces.

Among the many hormones produced by the pituitary gland are:

- Growth hormone, which aids in the body's processing of nutrients and minerals and promotes the development of bone and other bodily tissues.
- Prolactin, which is pronounced pro-LAK-tin, stimulates the production of milk in nursing mothers.
- Thyrotropin, which causes the thyroid gland to produce thyroid hormones, is pronounced thy-ruh-TRO-pin.
- corticotropin, which causes the adrenal gland to produce specific hormones (pronounced kor-tih-ko-TRO-pin).
- The hormone known as an antidiuretic (pronounced an-ty-dy-uh-REH-tik) regulates the body's water balance by acting on the kidneys.
- Oxytocin, which is pronounced "ahk-see-TOE-sin," is what causes the uterine contractions that occur during childbirth.

Endorphins (pronounced en-DOR-fins), which work on the neurological system and lessen pain perception, are also secreted by the pituitary. Hormones secreted by the pituitary also instruct the reproductive organs to produce sex hormones. In women, the pituitary gland also regulates the menstrual cycle and ovulation.

Thyroid: Located in the front portion of the lower neck, the thyroid is pronounced THY-royd. It has a butterfly or bow tie form. It produces the thyroid hormones triiodothyronine (pronounced try-eye-oh-doe-THY-ruh-neen) and thyroxine (pronounced thy-RAHK-sin). These hormones regulate how quickly cells burn food-based fuels to produce energy. The body's chemical reactions speed up with the amount of thyroid hormone in the blood.

Thyroid hormones are crucial for the growth and development of children's and adolescents' bones as well as for the development of the brain and nervous system.

The parathyroids are a group of four small glands that are connected to the thyroid. They are pronounced par-uh-THY-roydz. They release parathyroid hormone, which works with calcitonin (pronounced kal-suh-TOE-nin), which is produced by the thyroid, to regulate blood calcium levels.

Adrenal Glands: Perched atop each kidney are these two triangular adrenal glands (pronounced uh-DREE-nul). Each of the two components of the adrenal glands produces a distinct set of hormones and has a distinct purpose:

1. The adrenal cortex is the outer portion. It produces hormones known as corticosteroids (pronounced kor-tih-ko-STER-oydz), which aid in regulating the body's water and salt balance, metabolism, the immune system, stress response, and sexual development and function.
2. The adrenal medulla (pronounced muh-DUH-luh) is the inner portion. It produces catecholamines like epinephrine (pronounced eh-puh-NEH-frun) (pronounced kah-tuh-KO-luh-meenz). When the body is under stress, epinephrine, often known as adrenaline, raises heart rate and blood pressure.

Pineal: Located in the center of the brain is the pineal body, also known as the pineal gland (pronounced pih-NEE-ul). Melatonin (pronounced meh-luh-TOE-nin), a hormone that may assist control when you go to sleep at night and get up in the morning, is secreted by it.

Reproductive Glands: The primary source of sex hormones is the gonads. The majority of people are unaware that both men and women have gonads. In men, the testes, also known as the male gonads, are located in the scrotum. Testosterone (pronounced tess-TOSS-tuh-rone) is the most significant of the androgens (pronounced AN-druh-junz) that they secrete. These hormones alert a man's body to the onset of puberty-related changes, such as height and penis growth, a deeper voice, and the development of pubic and facial hair. Together with pituitary hormones, testosterone also signals to the body when a man's testes are ready to produce sperm.

The ovaries (pronounced OH-vuh-reez) are a girl's gonads, located in her pelvis. In addition to producing eggs, they release the feminine hormones progesterone (pronounced pro-JESS-tuh-rone) and estrogen (pronounced ESS-truh-jen). When a girl begins puberty, estrogen plays a part. A girl going through puberty will experience a growth spurt, breast development, and the beginning of body fat accumulation around the hips and thighs. The control of a girl's menstrual cycle is also influenced by estrogen and progesterone. These hormones are involved in pregnancy as well.

Pancreas: The hormones insulin (pronounced IN-suh-lin) and glucagon (pronounced GLOO-kuh-gawn), which regulate blood glucose (or sugar), are produced by the pancreas (pronounced PAN-kree-us). Insulin aids in maintaining the body's energy reserves. This stored energy helps organs function properly and is used by the body for activity and exercise.

How Can I Maintain the Health of My Endocrine System?

To maintain the health of your endocrine system:

- Make sure you exercise frequently.
- Consume a healthy diet.
- Get regular checks with your doctor.
- Before using any herbal remedies or supplements, see your doctor.
- Inform the physician of any family history of endocrine disorders, such as thyroid or diabetes.

Is It Time to Call the Doctor?

Inform the physician if you:

- Despite drinking plenty of water, you still feel thirsty.
- frequently need to urinate
- You experience nausea or stomach pain frequently.
- are weak or really exhausted.
- are significantly gaining or losing weight
- tremble or perspire a lot
- Are you constipated?
- are not developing or growing as anticipated.

The Reproductive System

What is the function of the reproductive system?

A man can conceive a woman and have her give birth thanks to the reproductive system, which is a network of organs and hormone production in both sexes. An egg cell in the woman and a sperm cell from the male combine during conception to form a fertilized egg, or embryo, which implants and develops in the uterus throughout pregnancy.

Infertility in both men and women is frequently caused by abnormalities or injury to the reproductive organs as well as malfunctions in the hormone production and delivery system that controls reproduction.

How the reproductive system's brain functions

The reproductive hormones and system are regulated and controlled in large part by brain areas. Chemical messengers known as hormones have an impact on the metabolism of other cells that have hormone receptors. To start an action, hormones can be made in one area of the body and then transported to another area through the blood.

The hypothalamus, which is situated in the center of the brain, and the pituitary gland, which is situated at the base of the brain, directly beneath the hypothalamus, make up the reproductive brain centers. The hypothalamus is influenced by activity in other higher brain areas.

To control the pituitary gland's synthesis and release of follicle-stimulating hormone (FSH) and luteinizing hormone (LH), the brain generates gonadotropin-releasing hormone (GnRH). The two gonadotropic hormones that are involved in both male and female reproduction are FSH and LH. The hypothalamus's GnRH pulses' amplitude and rate control the pituitary gland's production of FSH and LH.

Women's reproductive hormones

Hormones generated in the ovary, pituitary, and hypothalamus interact intricately to control the menstrual cycle. The pituitary's production of FSH encourages the ovarian follicles to start developing and maturing. The ovary contains sac-like structures called follicles that hold eggs. The follicle's cells generate estrogen as the follicle and egg grow. Inhibin, a different hormone produced by follicle cells, is sent back to the pituitary and hypothalamus to reduce the production of FSH.

As the follicle grows larger and matures, FSH continues to boost the amount of estrogen produced. The follicle produces its most estrogen as it reaches maturity, which causes the pituitary gland to release more LH quickly.

Together with the ovaries' production of estrogen, LH aids in the egg's maturation process. Ovulation, or the release of a mature egg from one of the ovary's follicles, is likewise triggered by LH. Following ovulation, the follicle transforms into the corpus luteum, a new tissue that makes progesterone.

In order to prepare for implantation, progesterone thickens the endometrium, the lining of the uterus. Pregnancy and implantation depend on progesterone. The thicker endometrium will disintegrate and disappear with menstrual flow if implantation is unsuccessful.

Male reproductive hormones

Spermatogenesis is the process by which the pituitary gland's FSH stimulates the testes to create sperm in men. Sperm maturation is aided by the pituitary gland's LH, which instructs the testes to create testosterone. The main sex hormone in men is testosterone.

Important roles and components of the reproductive system in women

The reproductive system of females is made to:

- Create the ova, also known as oocytes (ovum is singular for one egg), which are the eggs required for reproduction.
- A fertilized egg should be nurtured and incubated until it is fully developed.
- Generate the sex hormones for women that keep the reproductive cycle going.

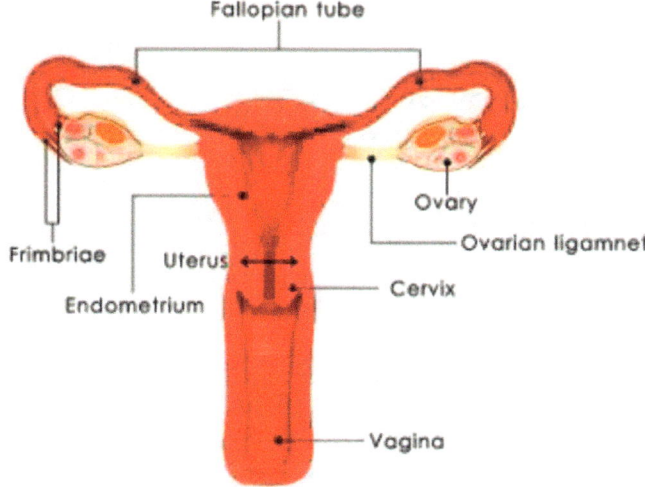

The reproductive organs of females consist of:

- **Ovaries:** On either side of the uterus are two tiny, oval-shaped glands known as the ovaries. They create the female sex hormone, estrogen, and house the female sex cells, known as eggs.
- **Fallopian tubes:** These are tiny passageways that a fertilized egg must go through in order to reach the uterus. Fertility issues can occasionally result from tubal disease, which includes damage or blockage to the fallopian tubes. Find out more about typical issues with fertility.
- **Uterus:** The uterus is a pear-shaped, hollow organ situated between the rectum and the bladder in a woman's lower abdomen. During pregnancy, the fetus is held in what is also known as the "womb." The uterus produces a nutrient-rich lining called the endometrium every month. This lining serves the reproductive function of feeding a growing fetus. By obstructing egg fertilization or the implantation and development of embryos, uterine abnormalities such fibroids or endometriosis can result in infertility.
- **Cervix** – The narrow, lower portion of the uterus between the rectum and bladder is called the cervix. It creates a passageway that leads to the vagina. The cervix, often known as the neck or the entrance to the womb, is where semen enters the uterus and menstrual blood exits. Polyps, which are growths in the cervix, can occasionally interfere with the process of fertilization or embryo development.

- **Vagina:** Also referred to as the birth canal, the vagina connects the cervix, or bottom portion of the uterus, to the external environment.
- **Vulva:** The exterior part of the female genital organs is called the vulva.

Important roles and components of the male reproductive system

The following tasks are carried out by the male reproductive system:

- Generates, preserves, and moves semen, the protective fluid, and sperm, the male reproductive cells.
- During intercourse, sperm are released into the female reproductive system.
- Generates and releases the sex hormones that keep the male reproductive system functioning.

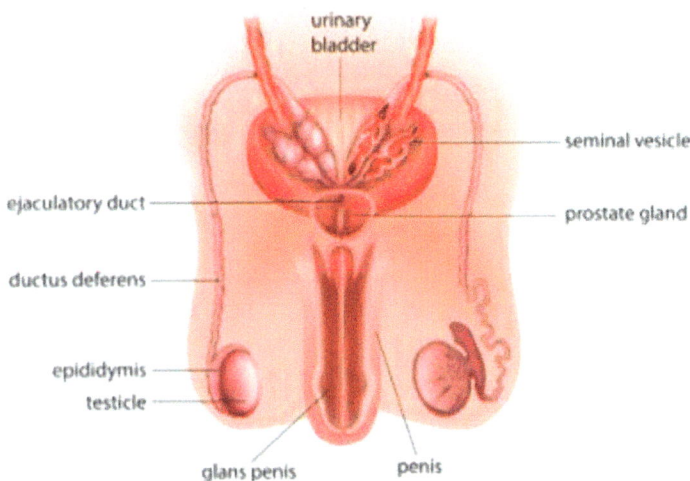

The majority of male reproductive organs are external, in contrast to the female reproductive system. Among them are:

- **Penis:** The shaft and the head are the two components that make up the penis. During sexual activity, sperm are delivered into the vagina through the urethral hole at the tip of the penis.
- **Skrotum**: The sac-like organ that hangs beneath and behind the penis is called the scrotum. Along with numerous nerves and blood vessels, it houses the testicles, sometimes known as the testes.
- **Testes (testes)** – The main male reproductive organ, the testes are oval organs located in the scrotum that produce sperm and testosterone.
- **Epididymis:** Located in the rear of each testicle, the epididymis is a C-shaped tube. Sperm cells generated in the testes are transported and stored by it. Since the sperm that emerge from the testes are immature and unable to fertilize, the epididymis also matures the sperm. Contractions push the sperm into the vas deferens during sexual stimulation.
- **Ductus (vas) deferens:** This lengthy, muscular tube is located right behind the bladder and extends from the epididymis into the pelvic cavity. In order to prepare for ejaculation, the vas deferens transports mature sperm to the urethra, the tube that transports pee or sperm outside of the body.

- **Ejaculatory ducts:** These are created when the seminal vesicles and vas deferens fuse together. The urethra is where the ejaculatory ducts empty.
- **Urethra:** Urine is transported from the bladder to the exterior of the body via the urethra. When a guy experiences sexual climax, it also has the added function of ejaculating semen. Only semen can be expelled at climax when the penis is erect during intercourse, blocking the flow of urine from the urethra.
- **Other glands:** To aid in reproduction, a number of glands generate fluid or semen. The fructose produced by the seminal vesicle gives the sperm energy while they search for an egg. Additionally, the prostate gland secretes a substance that facilitates the sperm's faster passage through the female reproductive system. A other group of glands known as bulbourethral, or occasionally Cowper's, glands produce a fluid that shields the sperm as they pass through the urethra.

Musculoskeletal System

The human body's musculoskeletal system, also known as the locomotor system, gives our bodies their structure, support, mobility, and stability. It is separated into two major categories:

- The body's muscular system, which consists of every kind of muscle. Movements are produced by the action of skeletal muscles, namely, on the joints of the body. The tendons that connect the muscles to the bones are also part of the muscular system.
- Skeletal system, in which bones are the primary constituent. Our bodies have a rigid yet flexible skeleton because of the way bones articulate with one another to form joints. The skeletal system's accessory structures—articular cartilage, ligaments, and bursae—support the integrity and functionality of the bones and joints.

The musculoskeletal system serves a variety of purposes beyond its primary role in giving the body stability and mobility. The skeletal portion is crucial for other homeostatic processes like hematopoiesis and the storage of minerals like calcium, while the muscular system stores most of the body's carbohydrates as glycogen.

You will learn about the musculoskeletal system's anatomy and function from this book.

Important information on the musculoskeletal system

Table quiz

Definition	A human body system that provides the body with movement, stability, shape, and support
Components	Muscular system: skeletal muscles and tendons Skeletal system: bones, joints; associated tissues (cartilage, ligaments, joint capsule, bursae)
Function	Muscles: Movement production, joint stabilization, maintaining posture, body heat production Bones: Mechanical basis for movements, providing framework for the body, vital organs protection, blood cells production, storage of minerals

The muscular system

Specialized contractile tissue known as muscle tissue makes up the muscular system, an organ system. All muscles are divided into three groups according to the three types of muscular tissue:

- The cardiac muscle, which makes up the myocardium, the heart's muscular layer
- Smooth muscle, which makes up hollow organs and blood vessel walls
- Skeletal muscle, which facilitates voluntary movement and is attached to the bones.

These types are divided into striated and non-striated muscles based on their histological appearance; smooth muscle is non-striated, whilst skeletal and cardiac muscles are categorized as striated. Since the skeletal muscles are innervated by the somatic portion of the nervous system, they are the only muscles that we can control with our will. On the other hand, the autonomic centers in our brains instinctively control the smooth and cardiac muscles since they are innervated by the autonomic nervous system.

The skeletal muscles

The primary functioning units of the muscular system are the skeletal muscles. The human body contains about 600 muscles. With the quadriceps femoris muscle in the leg being the largest and the stapedius muscle in the inner ear being the smallest, they differ drastically in size and structure.

For each part of the body, the skeletal muscles are arranged into one of four groups:

- The head and neck muscles, which comprise the pharyngeal, laryngeal, orbital, facial expression, masticatory, tongue, and neck muscles.
- The trunk muscles, which comprise the pelvic floor muscles, the back muscles, and the anterior and lateral abdominal muscles
- The upper limb muscles, which comprise the hand, arm, shoulder, and forearm muscles.

- Lower limb muscles, such as the muscles in the legs, feet, and hips and thighs

It can be overwhelming to realize that the body has over 600 muscles. Take a look at our simplified muscular anatomy reference charts if you're sick of large, detailed anatomy books. They provide all the information about muscles in one convenient location, arranged in tidy tables!

Structure

Fibers of muscles

Myofibra

1/6

Myocyte, Myofiber, show more are synonyms.

Myocytes, also known as muscle fibers or myofibrils, are the skeletal muscle cells that make up the skeletal muscles structurally. The primary characteristic of muscle fibers, which are specialized cells, is their capacity for contraction. The sarcolemma, a type of cell membrane, encloses these multinucleated, elongated, cylindrical cells. Sarcoplasm, the cytoplasm of skeletal muscle fibers, is home to contractile proteins such as myosin and actin. Sarcomeres are the units of contractile micro-apparatus made up of these proteins organized in patterns.

The endomysium is a loose sheath of connective tissue that envelops each muscle fiber. Muscle fascicles or muscle bundles are collections of many muscle fibers that are encased in a perimysium, a sheath of connective tissue. Finally, a collection of muscular fascicles makes up a complete muscle belly, which is encased on the outside by an additional layer of connective tissue known as the epimysium. The deep fascia of skeletal muscle, another layer of connective tissue that divides the muscles from other tissues and organs, is continuous with this layer.

Skeletal muscle tissue has four primary physiological characteristics because of its structure:

- Excitability: the capacity to recognize action potentials, which are brain stimuli;
- Contractibility: the capacity to contract in reaction to a signal from the brain;
- Extensibility: a muscle's capacity to stretch without rupturing;
- Elasticity: the capacity to regain its original shape following an extension.

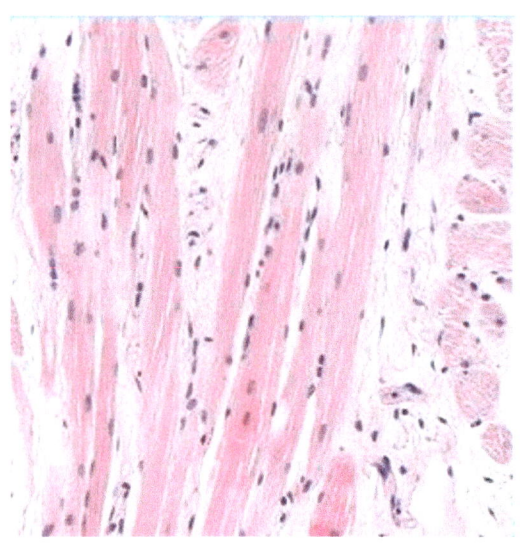

Skeletal muscle

Contraction of muscles

The ability of skeletal muscles to contract is their most crucial characteristic. The interaction of myofibrils within the muscle cells causes muscular contraction. This action creates a force that either speeds up or slows down a movement by shortening or tightening the muscle.

Muscle contractions can be classified as either isometric or isotonic. An isometric contraction is one in which the muscle's length does not vary during the contraction, while an isotonic contraction is one in which the tension does not change as the muscle's length does. Isotonic contractions come in two varieties:

- Concentric contraction, where the muscle shortens as a result of producing sufficient force to overcome the resistance. Any observable movement, like as lifting a barbell or walking up an incline, is made easier by this kind of contraction.
- Eccentric contraction, in which the muscle expands because the force it produces is less than the resistance. High tension is maintained by the muscle during an eccentric contraction. Typically, this kind of contraction is used to slow down a movement, like walking downhill or lowering a barbell.

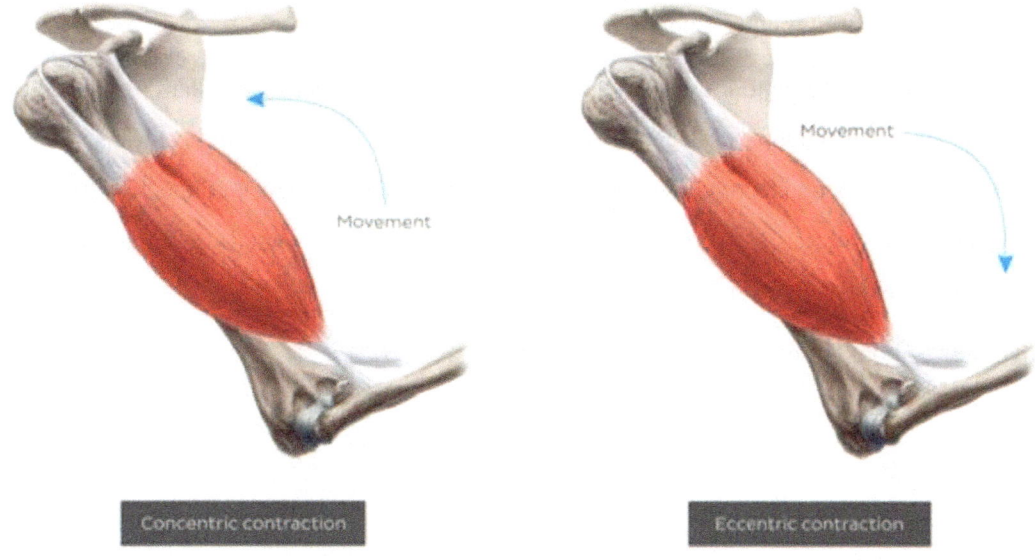

Muscle contractions that are eccentric and concentric (diagram)

Axon of a motor neuron

Axon motoneuri

1/2

No synonyms

The action potential, a signal produced by the nervous system, starts the chain of events that causes a muscle cell to contract. To get to the neuromuscular junction—the point where the motor nerve and muscle meet—this signal passes via motor neurons. The motor unit is a collection of muscle cells innervated by a single motor nerve's branches.

Acetylcholine (ACh) is released from the motor nerve into the synaptic cleft, which is the area between the sarcolemma and the nerve terminal, in response to the incoming action potential. The muscle cell undergoes a chemical process when the ACh attaches to the sarcolemma's receptors. This entails the sarcoplasmic reticulum releasing calcium ions, which in turn causes the muscle cell's contractile proteins to rearrange. Actin and myosin are the primary proteins involved; when ATP is present, they slide over one another and pull the ends of each muscle cell together to produce a contraction. The chemical reaction reverses and the muscle relaxes as the nerve signal weakens.

Tendons

Tendon

Tendo

1/5

No synonyms

Skeletal muscles are attached to bones by means of tendons, which are strong, pliable bands of thick connective tissue. Both the distal and proximal ends of muscles have tendon attachments, which connect them to the bone's periosteum at the proximal (origin) and distal attachments (insertion). Tendons pull the bones as muscles contract, transferring the mechanical force to the bones and resulting in movement.

The tendons' great tensile strength (resistance to longitudinal force) is a result of its dense, regular connective tissue and profusion of parallel collagen fibers. A tendon's collagen fibers are arranged into fascicles, and each fascicle is covered in an endotenon, a thin covering of thick connective tissue. In turn, a layer of dense, uneven connective tissue known as the epitenon surrounds clusters of fascicles. Lastly, a tiny band of connective tissue known as the mesotenon attaches to the epitenon, which is surrounded by a synovial sheath.

In this study unit, discover more about the microstructure of tendons:

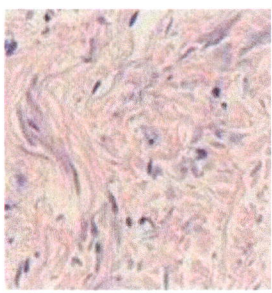

Study unit on dense connective tissue

The muscular system's functions

The muscular system's primary job is to generate bodily movement. The musculoskeletal system is capable of performing a variety of movements, depending on the axis and plane. Among the most significant ones are:

Leg flexion

Flexio cruris

1/8

Synonyms: knee flexion, genus Flexio

- Flexion and extension are movements in which the angle between the moving bones is decreased or increased, respectively. This movement revolves around a frontal axis in the sagittal plane. Bending the leg at the knee joint is an example of flexion, while straightening the knee from a flexed posture is an example of extension.
- Adduction and abduction are motions that move the body's components closer to or farther from the midline, respectively. These motions revolve around a sagittal axis in the frontal plane. For instance, moving the arm away from the side of the body is known as abduction at the shoulder joint, but bringing it back towards the body is known as adduction.
- In the transverse plane, rotation is the movement of a body part around its vertical (longitudinal) axis. Internal rotation is bringing the segment toward the midline, and external rotation is moving it away from the midline. This movement is defined in relation to the midline. The thigh's medial or lateral rotation are two examples.

- Two unique rotatory movement types that are frequently employed to characterize forearm movements are supination and pronation. In essence, supination is a lateral rotation of the forearm that causes the palms to spin superiorly when the elbow is flexed or anteriorly if the arm is in its natural position. These motions are also occasionally used to describe ankle and foot movements, where pronation refers to rolling the foot inward and supination to rolling the foot outward.

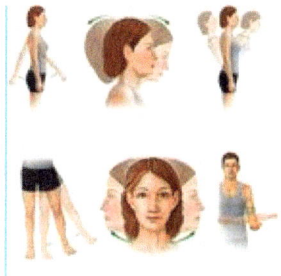

Body movement types: an exploration of the study unit

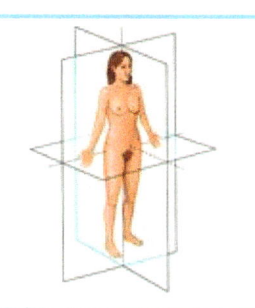

Explore the study unit using body planes and directional terminology.

Muscles support and stabilize joints generally, both when moving and when in a resting state. The articulating bones are stabilized and held in place by the passage of several muscles and their tendons over joints. Furthermore, the muscles are crucial for maintaining proper posture. The posture is maintained by a prolonged tonic contraction of postural muscles, even if the movements are mostly caused by muscles contracting and relaxing sporadically. When standing or walking, these muscles stabilize the body by acting against gravity. The back and abdominal muscles are part of the postural muscles.

Muscles also play a crucial role in producing heat. muscular tissue is one of the most metabolically active tissues in the body, in which roughly 85 percent of the heat produced in the body is the result of muscular contraction. Because of this, muscles are crucial for preserving a healthy body temperature.

Examine several frequently used roots, prefixes, and suffixes associated with the muscular system in order to enhance your knowledge of its vocabulary.

To what extent are you familiar with the body's major muscles? Take this quiz to see how much you know at a variety of levels of difficulty!

What is highlighted in green?

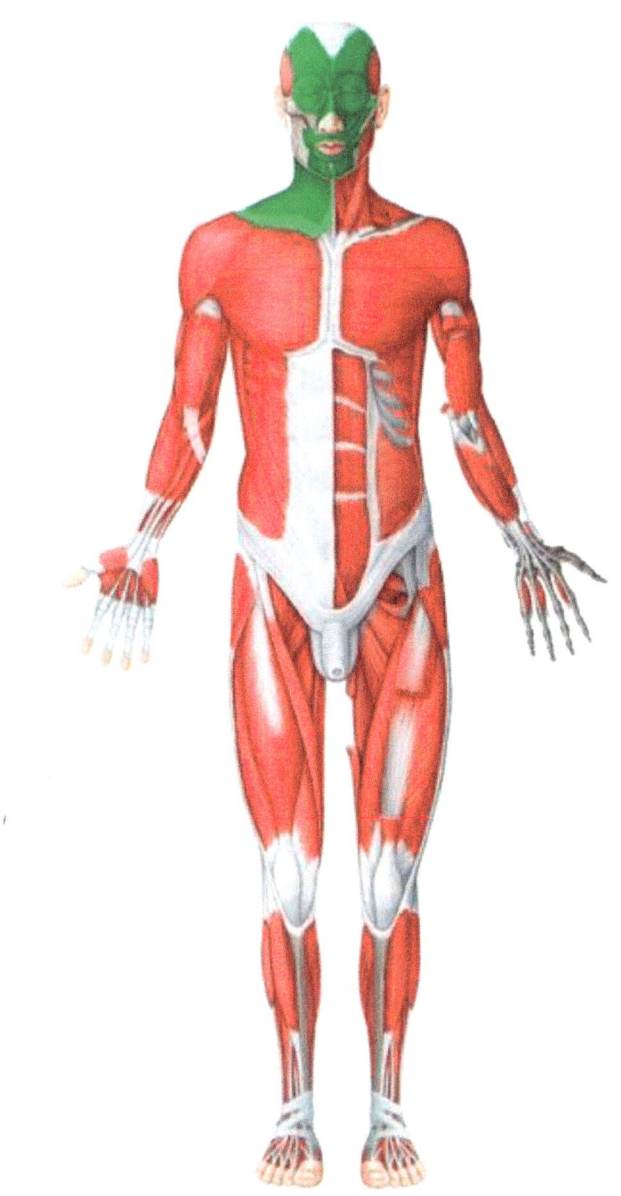

Facial expression muscles

Tongue muscles

Neck muscles

The back's superficial muscles

The skeletal system

The 206 bones and cartilages that make up the adult human skeleton. The bones are supported by ligaments, tendons, bursae, and muscles. The body's bones are arranged in two separate divisions:

- The bones that run down the body's long axis make up the axial skeleton. The vertebral column, head bones, and thoracic cage bones make up the axial skeleton.
- The appendicular skeleton, which includes the upper and lower extremity bones, the shoulder bones, and the pelvic girdle.

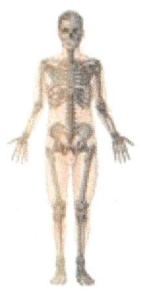

Skeletal system

Bones

Bone

Os

1/6

Systema skeletale and skeletal system are synonyms.

Dense, calcified connective tissue makes up the stiff structures known as bones. Type 1 collagen fibers scattered throughout the ground material make up the mineralized bone matrix that makes up bone tissue. Osteocytes, osteoblasts, and osteoclasts are three different types of specialized bone cells that make up the cellular component of bones.

The two separate layers that make up the bones have different histology features and appearances;

- The outer, denser layer of bone, known as compact (cortical) bone, is what gives the bone its smooth, solid, and white appearance. The periosteum is a layer of thick connective tissue that covers the compact bone's outside. The endosteum, which separates the compact and spongy bones, covers the inner surface of the compact bone.
- The deep, airy layer of the bone is called "spongy" (cancellous) bone. Spongy bone is more metabolically active and highly vascularized than compact bone. Usually, it is located in the vertebrae and at the extremities of long bones. The bone marrow, which is where adult hematopoiesis occurs, is located in the middle of spongy bone in some bones, such as the femur, sternum, or hip bone.

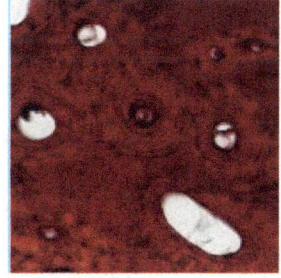

Bone Tissue

Bone types

Based on their forms, bones can be categorized as follows:

The humerus

1/5

No synonyms

- Long bones are tubular in shape, with a shorter transverse diameter and a longer longitudinal diameter. They are mostly made of compact bone, with the ends of the bones being filled with bony marrow and spongy bone. The clavicle, tibia, ulna, and humerus are a few examples of lengthy bones.
- The spongy bone in short bones is surrounded by a thin layer of compact bone, giving them a roughly cuboid or spherical form. The carpal and tarsal bones are two examples.
- Flat bones are typically bent, thin, and flattened. They have a layer of spongy bone encircled by two parallel layers of solid bones. Examples include the sacrum, sternum, scapula, and the majority of the skull bones.
- Where a muscle tendon crosses a joint, sesamoid bones—small, rounded, distinct bone types—are lodged in the tendon. Although the patella is the largest sesamoid bone in the body, the hand and foot have a number of smaller sesamoid bones, most of which are located around the joints.
- None of the other categories apply to irregular bones. Soft tissue and neurovascular structures typically pass through foramina found in uneven bones. The hip bone, vertebrae, and a few skull bones are a few examples.

On both its proximal and distal ends, a normal long bone has a long shaft (diaphysis) that extends into a neck (metaphysis) and head (epiphysis). Along with the attachment sites for ligaments and tendons, it also has a variety of markings and formations that allow passage for neurovascular structures. Among those characteristics are:

- Sulcus: a shallow groove on the surface of a bone (such as the humerus' radial sulcus).
- Condyle: a rounded articular region, such as the tibia's lateral condyle
- Epicondyle: prominence above a condyle (femur medial epicondyle)
- Crest: a bone ridge, such as the iliac crest
- A smooth, flat region that is typically covered in cartilage is called a facet (e.g. articular facet on vertebrae).
- A foramen is a passageway through a bone, such as the occipital bone's foramen magnum.

Cartilage

The hyaline cartilage

Hyalina Cartilago

1/7

No synonyms

A flexible connective tissue, cartilage is present in the body's various organ systems. Collagen fibers, specialized cells known as chondrocytes, and a plentiful ground substance that is high in proteoglycan and elastin fibers make up cartilage.

Based on its composition, cartilage is divided into the following types:

- Type II collagen and a large amount of pulverized substance make up hyaline cartilage, which gives it a shiny appearance. It is the most prevalent kind of cartilage in the nose, larynx, trachea, ribs, and joints (articular cartilage).
- Although it has more elastic fibers, elastic cartilage is comparable to hyaline cartilage. The auditory tube, the epiglottis, and the pinna of the ear are among the structures that contain it.
- A greater proportion of type I collagen fibers and a lesser quantity of ground substance make up fibrocartilage. Fibrocartilage is found in the pubic region, intervertebral discs, and various symphyses.

Articular cartilage, a form of cartilage that lines the articulating surfaces of bones, is specifically found in the musculoskeletal system. The articulating bones can bear weight and move over one another with minimal friction thanks to the articular cartilage, which also gives them congruence.

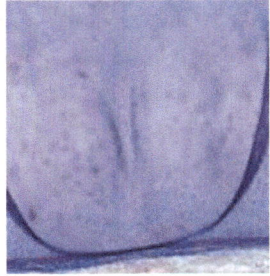

Hyaline Cartilage Exploration

Joints

Every musculoskeletal bone is joined to one or more other bones by a joint. The bones pivot on the joints, which give them a fulcrum, enabling body parts to move. However, some joints, including those between the skull's bones, do not move, therefore this is not a necessary feature of a joint. Bony congruence and structures that cross the joint, including ligaments and tendons, are two of the many components that provide a joint its stability and integrity.

Joints can be divided into the following categories according to the range of mobility they display and the kind of tissue that keeps the nearby bones together:

- Synovial joints are freely moving joints where the synovial cavity, a possible gap between the bones, separates them rather than putting them in direct touch. The synovial fluid, which lubricates and nourishes the articulating surfaces to lessen friction, is secreted by the synovial membrane lining the synovial cavity. Hyaline cartilage lines the articulating bones in the majority of synovial joints. The joint capsule, supporting ligaments, and muscles that traverse the joint all contribute to the typical wide range of motion of these joints. The sternoclavicular, elbow, shoulder, and knee joints are examples of synovial joints.
- The articulations where the bones are joined by thick fibrous connective tissue are known as fibrous joints. Fibrous joints provide very little movement since the bones are securely bound together. The cuboideonavicular joints, distal tibiofibular joints, and the cranial sutures are all fibrous joints.

- Cartilaginous joints are articulations where cartilage connects the bones. Between synovial and fibrous joints, the bones can move. Cartilaginous joints can be classified as either symphysis joints (like the pubic symphysis) or synchondrosis joints (like the costochondral joints).

Joint of the ball and socket

Speacular Articulation

1/5

Cotyloid joint, spheroidal joint, and more are synonyms.

The synovial joints can be further classified into six main categories based on the movements they permit and/or the form of their articulating surface:

- The hip joint is an example of a ball and socket joint.
- Metacarpophalangeal joints are examples of condyloid joints.
- Elbow joints, for example, are hinge joints.
- Atlanto-axial joints, for example, are pivot joints.
- Saddle joints (carpometacarpal joint, for example)
- Acromioclavicular joints, for example, are plane joints.

Ligaments

Ligaments resemble tendons in structure and are fibrous bands composed of thick regular connective tissue. The ligaments join bone to bone, as opposed to the tendons that join muscles to bone. Ligaments are present in many other areas of the body outside the musculoskeletal system, where they typically transport neurovascular systems and maintain and hold internal organs in place.

The iliofemoral ligament

Iliofemoral Ligamentum

1/5

Bigelow's Y-ligament and Bertin's Ligament are synonyms.

Ligaments strengthen the joints and stabilize the articulating bones in the musculoskeletal system. Ligaments are divided into the following categories based on their anatomical location in relation to the joint capsule:

- In essence, capsular ligaments are thickenings of the joint capsule that take the shape of triangles or lengthy bands. The integrity of the joint capsule is strengthened by these ligaments. The iliofemoral ligament of the hip joint is an illustration of the capsular ligament.
- The ligaments that are located inside the joint capsule are known as intracapsular ligaments. Although they permit a significantly greater range of motion than other ligaments, these ligaments strengthen the bond between the joint's articulating surfaces. The anterior and posterior cruciate ligaments of the knee joint are two examples.

- Ligaments that are located outside the joint capsule are known as extracapsular ligaments. These ligaments are crucial for avoiding dislocations because they give the articulating bones the greatest stability. Extracapsular ligaments may be located near the joint capsule (such as the medial collateral ligament of the ankle joint) or slightly farther away (such as the vertebral ligaments).

The Bursae

Bursa suprapatellar

The suprapatellaris bursa

No synonyms

The synovial membrane lines the joint cavity's bursae, which are tiny sac-like outpouchings. They are present surrounding the joints, minimizing friction between neighboring components and cushioning the corresponding bones, tendons, and muscles.

Near the big joints of the arms and legs are most of the synovial bursae. One of the bursae of the knee joint, for instance, is the suprapatellar bursa, which is situated between the femur and the tendon of the quadriceps femoris muscle, superior to the patella. During knee flexion and extension, these structures can glide over one another without encountering any resistance because to the suprapatellar bursa.

It's time to sort out your skeletal system with our integrated quiz!

What is highlighted in green?

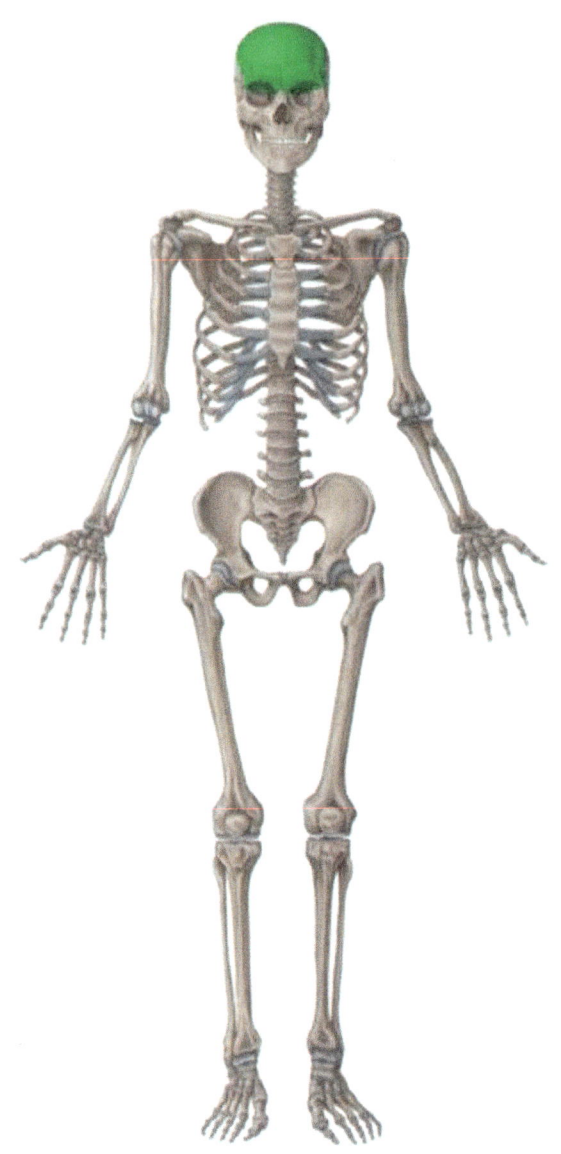

The frontal bone

The temporal bone

Maxilla

The mandible

The skeletal system's functions

There are several purposes for the skeletal system. The bones provide the body its structure and serve as the points where cartilage, muscles, tendons, and ligaments can join. Together, these tissues provide a force that serves as the biomechanical foundation for movement.

Because of its structural integrity, the skeletal system shields the internal organs, including the heart and lungs, which are shielded by the rib cage, and the brain, which is encased in the skull.

The skeletal system also performs a number of metabolic tasks. Important minerals, including calcium and phosphorus, are stored in the bones. Because of this, bones are necessary for maintaining blood calcium levels, which are controlled by varying the rate of bone resorption.

Finally, hematopoiesis, the process of creating new blood cells, takes place in the bone marrow found in spongy bone. Red blood cells, platelets, and white blood cells including monocytes, granulocytes, and lymphocytes are all made in the bone marrow.

We developed a unique summary test that covers the anatomy and histology of the musculoskeletal system's key components. You can customize this quiz by changing and filtering specific structures!

Clinical association

Numerous disorders can impact the joints, muscles, and bones. Musculoskeletal disorders can range from illnesses to mild physical impairments. Some clinical problems of the musculoskeletal system include the following:

Osteoporosis

"Porous bones" is the literal definition of osteoporosis, a disorder that weakens bones. This disorder causes the bones to become brittle and brittle, increasing the risk of fractures compared to healthy bones. Because of this, even a small bump or mishap can result in severe fractures.

The "bone of the old," particularly in women, is osteoporosis. Calcium is necessary for bone to be firm and rock-like. Bones lose density and become more brittle when too much calcium is dissolved from them or not enough is replenished. The female sex hormone estrogen aids in preserving healthy calcium levels in bones. Women are more likely to develop osteoporosis once the ovaries stop generating the hormone. A collapse of the spinal column's bony vertebrae causes stooped posture and a loss of height. Hip fractures happen often.

Sarcopenia

A progressive and widespread loss of skeletal muscle mass and strength is the hallmark of sarcopenia, a sickness that carries a risk of negative consequences like physical disability, a reduced quality of life, and even mortality.

The condition of arthritis

A collection of disorders affecting the joints is called arthritis. These disorders harm the joints, which typically leads to aging-related pain and stiffness. Almost every joint in the body, as well as numerous joint components, can be impacted by arthritis.

As people age, their joint tissues begin to degrade and lose their ability to withstand wear and tear. Swelling, discomfort, and frequently a lack of joint mobility are the symptoms of this degeneration. Osteoarthritis is a disorder in which the articulating bones and soft tissues of the joints change. Rheumatoid arthritis is a more severe type of the condition. The latter is an autoimmune condition in which the body creates antibodies that attack the tissues of the joints, leading to persistent inflammation, severe joint damage, pain, and immobility.

Dystrophia of the muscles

A class of muscle disorders known as muscular dystrophy impairs movement and weakens the musculoskeletal system. Progressive skeletal muscle weakening, abnormalities in muscle proteins, and the degeneration of muscle fibers (muscle cells) and tissue are the hallmarks of muscular dystrophies.

It is a collection of hereditary illnesses where the muscles that govern mobility gradually deteriorate. The root -trophy indicates to preserve normal nourishment, structure, and function, while the word dys- means aberrant. Duchenne muscular dystrophy is the most prevalent type in children and only affects boys. Those who are affected normally live into their late teens or early 20s, and it usually manifests between the ages of 2 and 6.

The following are additional musculoskeletal conditions:

- Erythematous lupus
- Myasthenia gravis
- Rotator cuff tear
- Tendonitis
- Carpal tunnel syndrome
- Osteomalacia

Nervous System

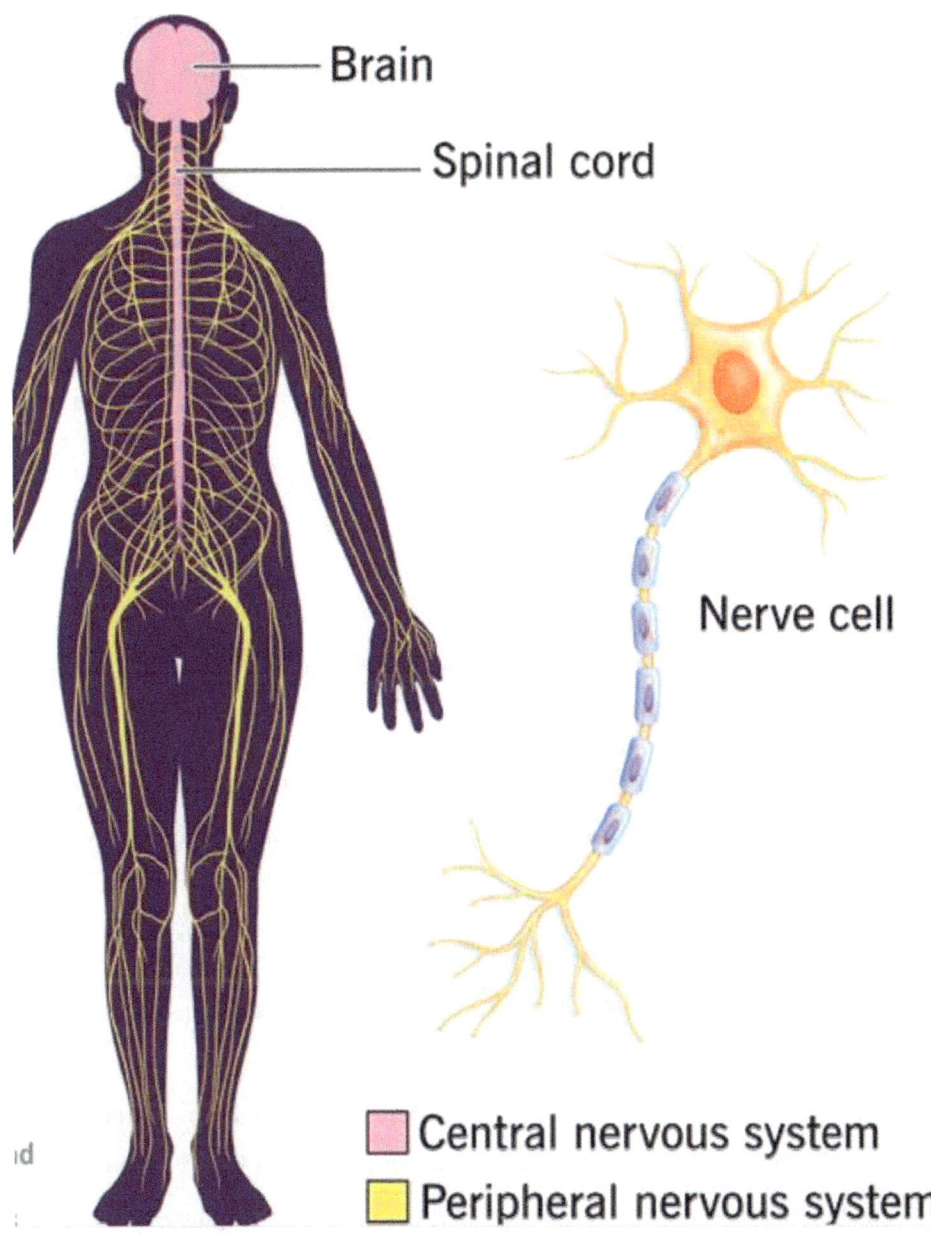

Your brain, spinal cord, and nerves are all part of your nervous system.

What is the nervous system?

Your body's command center is your nervous system. It is composed of your nerves, spinal cord, and brain. Electrical impulses, or messages, are sent from your brain to every other area of your body by your nervous system. For instance, these signals instruct you to speak, move, breathe, and see. Your nervous system monitors both internal and external events and determines how to react in every given circumstance.

Complex functions like memory and cognitive processes are controlled by your nervous system. It is also crucial for the automatic bodily functions including blushing, perspiration, and blinking.

Operation

What is the function of the nervous system?

The primary job of your nervous system is to transmit signals from your body's various components to your brain, which then relays those messages back to your body to instruct it on what to do. These messages control your:

- Feelings, learning, memory, and thoughts.
- Motions (coordination and balance).
- Senses (the way your brain processes what you touch, taste, hear, see, and feel).
- The healing of wounds.
- Rest.
- Patterns of breathing and heartbeat.
- The production of perspiration in response to stressful circumstances.
- Digestion.
- Physical changes like aging and puberty.

What is the nervous system's mechanism?

To transmit information, or messages, throughout your body, the nervous system employs nerve cells called neurons. Your muscles, glands, organs, skin, and brain all exchange these electrical signals.

You can move your limbs and experience pain and other sensations thanks to the communications. Information about your surroundings is taken in by your eyes, hearing, tongue, nose, and the nerves throughout your body. Nerves then transport that information to and from your brain.

Neurons come in various varieties. Every kind of neuron has a distinct function:

- Your brain and spinal cord send impulses to your muscles through motor neurons. They facilitate your mobility. Additionally, they help with speech, swallowing, and breathing.
- Your brain receives information from your senses—what you see, touch, taste, etc.—through sensory neurons.
- Motor and sensory neurons exchange information with one another. These neurons affect how you learn, think, and remember. They also control how you move in reaction to sensory input, such as avoiding hot surfaces.

The anatomy

Which components make up the nervous system?

There are two primary components to the nervous system:

- Central nervous system (CNS): The CNS is composed of the brain and spinal cord. To control your thoughts, movements, and emotions, your brain interprets messages from your nerves.
- Peripheral nervous system (PNS): A network of nerves makes up your PNS. Your spinal cord is the starting point for the nerves. Your arms, legs, fingers, toes, and organs all receive information from your brain and spinal cord through this system.

The peripheral nerve system is divided into two parts:

- Your voluntary motions are controlled by the somatic nervous system.
- Your unconscious actions (involuntary movements) are controlled by the autonomic nervous system.

What is the appearance of the nervous system?

The foundation of your nervous system is made up of nerve cells, or neurons. Your brain contains 100 billion neurons. All of your body's cells are connected.

Consider the nervous system to be a tree. Your brain and spinal cord are located in the trunk of your central nervous system. Your peripheral nervous system (nerves) are represented by the tree branches. The brain and spinal cord, which are the truck's branches, reach every region of your body.

Disorders and Conditions

Which common illnesses or conditions impact the neurological system?

Your nervous system might be affected by a variety of disorders. Among the most prevalent are:

- Alzheimer's illness.
- Cancer.
- Cerebral palsy.
- Epilepsy.
- Huntington's illness.
- Meningitis, an infection.
- Parkinson's illness.
- A stroke.
- Brain damage from trauma.

What are typical indications of disorders of the neurological system?

Nervous system disorders can present with a variety of signs and symptoms, such as:

- Modifications to coordination and movement.
- Loss of memory.
- Numbness, pain, or a tingling sensation.
- Modifications in mood and behavior.
- Thinking and reasoning difficulties.
- Fits.

A stroke is an example of a medical emergency that requires prompt attention. Get in touch with 911 or your local emergency services number if you observe any of the following symptoms:

- One side of your body may have paralysis or weak muscles.
- Abrupt loss of vision.
- Speech slurred.

- Perplexity.

Which tests evaluate your nervous system's health?

One of the following tests could be used by a medical professional to assess the condition of your neurological system:

- A CT scan, or computed tomography.
- EKG, or electrocardiogram.
- EEG, or electroencephalogram.
- Lumbar puncture, often known as spinal tap.
- MRI scans, or magnetic resonance imaging.

How are disorders of the neurological system managed?

In order to identify and treat any disorders affecting your nervous system, a medical professional will examine your symptoms. Every illness has a different course of treatment. In order to develop your treatment plan, your healthcare professional will examine a number of criteria, including your age and overall health. This strategy could consist of:

- Taking prescription drugs.
- Getting surgery.
- Taking part in therapy to receive emotional and mental assistance.
- Getting supportive care to ensure your comfort.

Care

How can I maintain the health of my neurological system?

You can maintain the health of your nervous system by:

- Routinely visiting a medical professional.
- Preserving health (e.g., by eating a balanced diet).
- Steering clear of dangerous chemicals, such as tobacco use.
- Donning protective gear, such as a helmet, when engaging in specific activities or sports.

Taking care of any underlying medical issues.

When should I contact a medical professional?

Make immediate contact with a healthcare professional if you observe any unexpected changes in your health, such as:

Weakness of muscles.

- Severe headaches or vision issues.
- Speech slurred.
- Your arms or legs may become numb, tingly, or lose their feeling.
- Tremors or tics, which are erratic muscle contractions.
- A shift in memory or behavior.
- Issues with muscle movement or coordination.

Call 911 or your local emergency services number if you or a loved one exhibits symptoms of a seizure or stroke.

A message

Your entire body is controlled by your neurological system. It facilitates thought, learning, movement, and memory. Your organs, muscles, and glands are all connected by this extensive network of nerves. It must be maintained in order to function. Your nervous system may occasionally be impacted by unforeseen circumstances, such as an infection, trauma, or underlying illness. A medical professional can help you maintain your health so that your nervous system has what it needs to operate normally.

Hematology oncology

Hematology oncology: what is it?

The medical disciplines of hematology, which studies blood, and oncology, which studies and treats cancer, are combined in hematology oncology.

Blood malignancies and blood-related illnesses are diagnosed, treated, and prevented by hematologic oncologists. The hematologic oncologists at City of Hope advanced medicines and a variety of diagnostic techniques, including imaging and laboratory tests offer patients with malignant hematologic disorders, such as

- leukemia
- multiple myeloma
- Hodgkin lymphoma
- non-Hodgkin lymphoma

Hematologic malignancies are distinct from other forms of cancer in that they may not develop into tumors and instead arise in the body's blood cells. The majority of hematologic oncologists do not handle operable cancers like lung or breast cancer, however some are skilled in treating solid tumors.

At City of Hope, hematology/oncology doctors undertake stem cell transplantation, a therapy option for some blood malignancies. Hematopoietic progenitor cell transplantation is another name for stem cell transplantation.

Together, City of Hope® and Cancer Treatment Centers of America® (CTCA) are extending patient access to comprehensive, individualized cancer care.

A hematologic oncologist would see a patient for what reason?

If a blood test reveals any abnormalities, patients may be referred to a hematologic oncologist. Red blood cells transport oxygen from the lungs to the heart and other organs, platelets clot blood and stop uncontrollable bleeding, white blood cells combat infection, and plasma transports waste products to the liver and kidneys.

A hematologic oncologist may look for indications of blood cancer or other blood abnormalities if a blood test shows an excess or deficiency of any of these blood components. For example, multiple myeloma can form in bone marrow plasma, whereas Hodgkin lymphoma and non-Hodgkin lymphoma develop in white blood cells called lymphocytes.

How are blood malignancies treated by hematologic oncologists?

A patient's age, the type of cancer they have, the rate at which the cancer is spreading, and other factors all affect how they are treated for blood cancer.

A comprehensive care team at City of Hope treats patients with blood cancer, aiming to eradicate the hematologic malignancies and lower the risk of recurrence. To keep the patient resilient, lessen treatment adverse effects, and preserve quality of life, the team may also provide supportive care.

The hematologic oncologist will create a thorough treatment plan in collaboration with the other members of the cancer care team, which may involve the following therapies.

- Immunotherapy, CAR T-cell treatment;
- chemotherapy;
- radiation therapy;
- targeted therapy;
- stem cell transplantation

The City of Hope cancer care team may suggest a variety of supportive care services, including pain management, psychosocial counseling, physical therapy, nutritional and/or naturopathic assistance, and others, to help minimize or prevent treatment side effects and hasten recovery.

What steps are involved in a stem cell transplant?

Patients now enjoy more advantages and fewer complications as a result of advances in stem cell research. Bone marrow, circulating (peripheral) blood, or umbilical cord blood are the sources of healthy stem cells. After that, the body receives an intravenous infusion of these blood-forming stem cells to replace any damaged or diseased bone marrow. The location of the healthy stem cell harvest determines the type of stem cell transplantation:

- Allogeneic stem cell transplants employ stem cells derived from a compatible donor, while autologous stem cell transplants use stem cells extracted from the patient's own body.
- Stimulating fresh bone marrow growth, suppressing the disease, and lowering the risk of relapse are the objectives of transplantation.

Before receiving a transplant, patients go through a conditioning program. This treatment plan seeks to eradicate as many cancer cells as possible, frequently by administering strong dosages of radiation or chemotherapy.

The patient's blood levels will be monitored by the care team for several months after the transplant, and they may recommend platelet and red blood cell transfusions if necessary.

The stem cell transplant teams at City of Hope hospitals across the United States collaborate with patients to meet their needs at every stage of the stem cell transplant procedure in order to lower the risk of problems and adverse effects.

Dermatologists

Dermatologists are medical professionals who focus on identifying and treating conditions affecting the skin, mucous membranes, hair, and nails. Surgeons can also be dermatologists.

A dermatologist: what is it?

The largest and heaviest organ in your body, your skin serves a variety of vital purposes. It shields you from harmful substances, pathogens, and extremes of temperature. Additionally, it's an excellent gauge of your general health because variations in the tone or texture of your skin may indicate a health issue. It's critical to know the general condition of your skin and to take appropriate care of it.

A dermatologist is a medical professional who specializes in treating conditions.

- skin
- Hair.
- Nails.

In addition to managing cosmetic conditions including scarring and hair loss, they are specialists in the diagnosis and treatment of diseases affecting the skin, hair, and nails.

What is the job of a dermatologist?

Skin disorders are diagnosed and treated by dermatologists. They are also able to identify skin symptoms that could be signs of internal issues, such as organ failure or disease.

Dermatologists frequently carry out specific diagnostic tests for skin disorders. Among the therapies they employ are:

- Injectable or externally administered medications.
- Light therapy using ultraviolet (UV) light.
- A variety of dermatological surgical procedures, including skin biopsies and mole removal; • Cosmetic operations, including laser treatments, sclerotherapy, and chemical peels.

What education and credentials are required of dermatologists?

Physicians must finish four years of schooling in order to become dermatologists.

- A four-year medical school program.
- A year-long internship that includes instruction in dermatology and other disciplines.
- Three years of residency, which is ongoing education focused on dermatology.
- One to two fellowship years. Although it is not required, a fellowship provides more training in a specialism of dermatology.
- Certification and licensing. Dermatologists must pass a board certification exam administered by the American Board of Dermatology, the American Osteopathic Board of Dermatology, or the Royal College of Physicians and Surgeons of Canada in order to be licensed to practice medicine in the United States.

Which conditions are frequently treated by dermatologists?

A dermatologist may treat a number of common ailments, such as:

- Eczema;
- Acne.
- Loss of hair.
- Fungus on the nails.
- Psoriasis.
- Skin cancer.
- Rosacea.

What kinds of operations do dermatologists carry out?

Typical practices consist of:

- **Electrosurgery:** This technique uses a high-frequency electric current to cut or destroy tissue during surgery.
- **Cryosurgery:** This technique uses extremely low temperatures to freeze and destroy tissue.
- **Laser surgery:** Using specific light beams for surgical purposes is known as laser surgery.
- **Excision surgery:** This procedure entails removing tissue with the proper closures by cutting it with a sharp knife, such as a scalpel.
- **Mohs surgery:** The medical procedure known as Mohs surgery entails removing cancer cells from your skin layer by layer.
- **Mole removal:** This procedure is removing a mole from your body, either completely or partially. They check the mole for skin conditions like malignancy.
- **Vein treatment:** Dermatologists may use laser or sclerotherapy to treat your damaged veins after assessing them.

What are some subspecialties within dermatology?

subspecialties in dermatology.

- Mohs surgery
- dermatopathology
- Dermatology in children.
- Dermatology that is cosmetic.

What distinguishes dermatologists from estheticians?

Medical professionals are not aestheticians. They are unable to prescribe drugs or diagnose skin conditions. Only therapies that alter your skin's look can benefit from their assistance. The following are a few esthetician procedures:

- Skin exfoliation, or scrub.
- Teaching students how to cover up scars with cosmetics.
- Using acne remedies.
- Making recommendations for skin care items.
- Waxing.

- Airbrush tanning.

When is the best time for me to see a dermatologist?

The following are some of the more typical symptoms that might warrant a visit to a dermatologist:

- The size, color, or shape of a mole or skin patch has changed.
- Skin cancer.
- Acne that is severe or persistent.
- Rash.
- Hives.
- Scars.
- Eczema.
- Psoriasis.
- Rosacea.
- Dark patches (hyperpigmentation) on your face.
- Prolonged inflammation of the skin.
- Infections.
- Warts.
- Loss of hair.
- Disorders of the nails.
- Age-related symptoms.
- Spider veins and varicose veins.

How should I get ready for my first visit to the dermatologist?

It's good to prepare for your first dermatologist visit in order to maximize its benefits. One option is to bring a list of the most crucial topics you wish to cover with your dermatologist.

- Take note of any modifications to your general health.
- Maintain a symptom notebook (and carry it with you) and note all of your occurrences, including the day, time, duration, intensity, triggers, symptoms, and any steps you take to put an end to the episode. If at all possible, bring crisp pictures.
- Find out about the medical history of your family. Your dermatologist can make an accurate diagnosis with the use of this information.
- To make it easier for your dermatologist to examine you, dress comfortably.
- Steer clear of nail polish and makeup. Your dermatologist may find it challenging to adequately inspect your skin or nails if you are wearing cosmetics or nail polish.
- Take into consideration circling areas of your body with a washable pen. You can better recall what to discuss with your dermatologist if you have physical reminders.

- Bring copies of all test findings, including pictures and lab work that were ordered from medical professionals outside of your dermatologist's network.
- Bring a list of every product you now use or take. Incorporate over-the-counter (OTC) and prescription drugs, vitamins, supplements, herbal products, soaps, sunscreens, and cosmetics. Additionally, inform your dermatologist of any past drug interactions or negative effects.
- Bring a list of the allergies you are aware of.
- Bring a friend or family member to the appointment to help with note-taking and to provide additional eyes and ears. In addition to asking questions and reminding you to schedule testing and follow-up appointments, this individual can assist in reviewing the conversation you had with your dermatologist.
- Find out whether you need to make another appointment to talk about any other issues.

A message

Physicians that specialize in skin, hair, and nails are known as dermatologists. Cosmetic conditions including scarring and hair loss are also treated by dermatologists. After examining you and ordering laboratory testing, your dermatologist will diagnose you and treat your condition with either medication or surgery. If necessary, they might collaborate with and refer you to another professional. Make notes and arrange your medical records before to your meeting. Make sure to inquire about anything that comes to mind. Your dermatologist wants to support you, assist you in diagnosing your illness, and treat or manage it as best they can.

Section 3

Clinical Presentations

General Approach to the Patient

The purpose of the medical interview is multifaceted. 1. It is employed to gather data to help with diagnosis (the "history" of the current illness), comprehend patient values, evaluate and convey prognosis, build a therapeutic alliance, and come to a consensus with the patient regarding additional diagnostic tests and treatment alternatives. Additionally, it provides a chance to affect patient behavior, for example, through encouraging conversations about quitting smoking or taking medications as prescribed. Patient satisfaction and involvement in care are increased by interviewing strategies that prevent the doctor from controlling the conversation. Health outcomes can be enhanced by improved patient involvement and efficient clinician-patient communication.

ADHERENCE OF PATIENTS

Successful prevention and treatment of many illnesses rely on challenging basic behavioral adjustments, such as changing one's diet, exercising, quitting smoking, reducing alcohol use, wearing masks to prevent infection, and following complicated prescription schedules. Every practice has issues with adherence; one-third of patients never take their medications, and up to 50% of patients do not follow to their treatment plans completely. Even those who have access to care, many people with health issues may not seek the right care or may discontinue treatment too soon. The number of interventions, their complexity and cost, and the patient's feeling of overmedication are all negatively connected with adherence rates for short-term, self-administered therapies, which are greater than those for long-term therapies.

For instance, adherence to antiretroviral therapy is a critical factor in determining the efficacy of treatment for people with HIV. Research has clearly shown that plasma HIV RNA levels, CD4 cell counts, and mortality are closely related to patient adherence. More than 95% adherence is required to sustain virologic suppression. Nonetheless, research indicates that adherence tends to decline over time and that 40% of patients are less than 90% adherent.

Simple forgetfulness, being away from home, being busy, and altering daily routine are some of the patient's causes for inadequate adherence. Additional factors include mental health conditions (such as substance abuse or depression), treatment adverse effects, regimen complexity, and doubt over the efficacy of treatment. Adherence has become even more challenging, especially for individuals with lower means, due to the rising costs of prescriptions, including generic drugs, and the increased burden of patient cost-sharing.

Patients appear to be more adept at taking their prescription drugs than following advice to alter their diet, exercise routine, alcohol consumption, or other self-care practices (such checking their blood sugar levels at home). Giving explicit instructions can enhance medication adherence for short-term regimens. It could be beneficial to put patient recommendations in writing, including medication adjustments. Due to the prevalence of inadequate functional health literacy (almost half of US patients who speak English cannot read and comprehend...

Why are symptoms and indicators important?

The terms "sign" and "symptom" can be used interchangeably. But a sign is something a doctor or other person observes, but a symptom is something a person experiences.

Although signs and symptoms are sometimes confused, there are significant distinctions between them that influence how they are used in medicine. A skin rash or cough are examples of objective signs of an illness. These can be recognized by a physician, a family member, and the person exhibiting the symptoms.

Less evident disruptions in regular functioning, like weariness, lower back discomfort, and stomachaches, are symptoms that only the individual experiencing them can identify. Because symptoms are subjective, others are only aware of them if the person with the disorder tells them.

Quick facts about symptoms and indicators

- Since no one else can see a mild headache, it can only ever be a symptom.
- There are three types of medical symptoms: remitting, relapsing, and chronic.
- High blood pressure, which can be measured and seen by another person, is an example of a medical indicator. In 1674,
- Anthony van Leuwenhoek created the microscope, which fundamentally altered the nature of diagnostic instruments.

Symptom versus sign

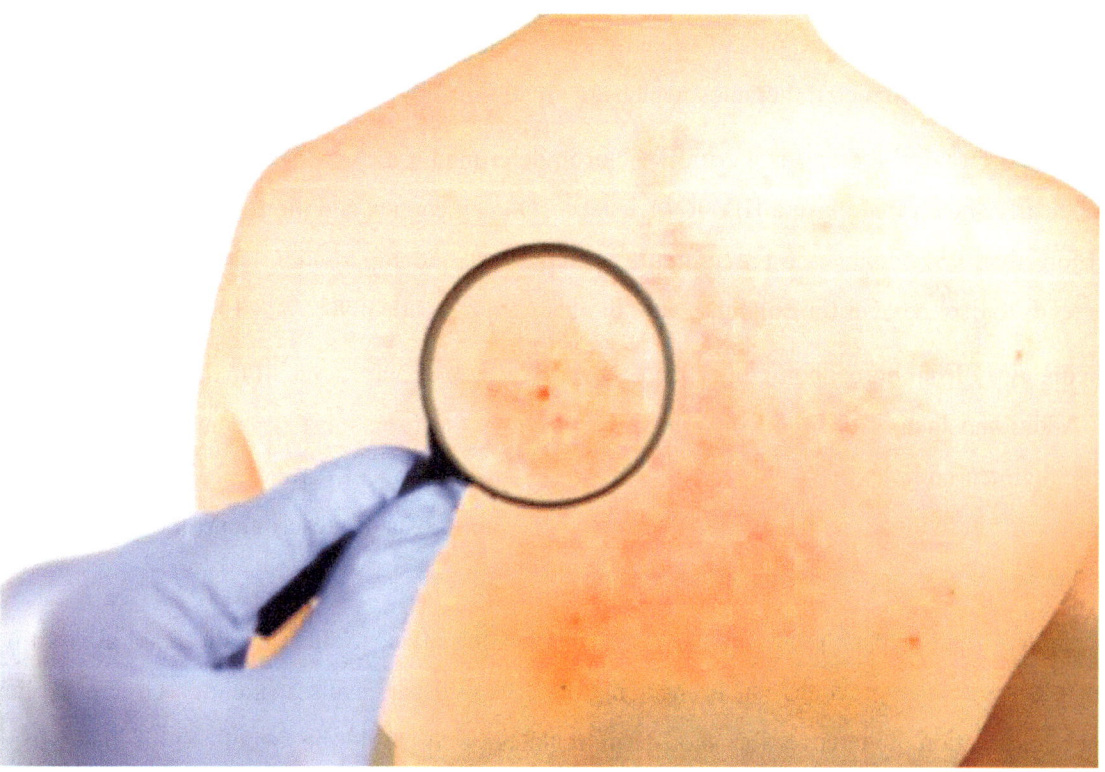

A sign is the result of a health issue that another person can see. A symptom is an impact that only the person with the ailment can see and feel.

Who sees the consequence is the primary distinction between signs and symptoms.

A rash, for instance, may be a symptom, a sign, or both:

- The rash is a symptom if the patient notices it, and a sign if the physician, nurse, or another person notices it.
- The rash may be considered both a sign and a symptom if both the patient and the physician observe it.

Signs and symptoms are the body's methods of alerting a person that something is amiss, regardless of who observes that a system or body component is not operating regularly. While some symptoms may go away entirely on their own without medical intervention, others require follow-up care.

History

Since Hippocrates required a patient's urine to be tasted, the identification of symptoms and indicators has advanced significantly.

As time and technology have advanced, the doctor's ability to recognize signals has become more and more crucial.

The ability to detect disease symptoms that are imperceptible to the human eye was made possible by Antony van Leeuwenhoek's invention of the microscope and its application in the 1674 discovery of cells and microorganisms. These include alterations in the makeup of waste products and blood, the presence of foreign organisms in the urine and blood, and other significant, microscopic indicators.

These markers have the power to distinguish between harmful illnesses and disorders and regular function.

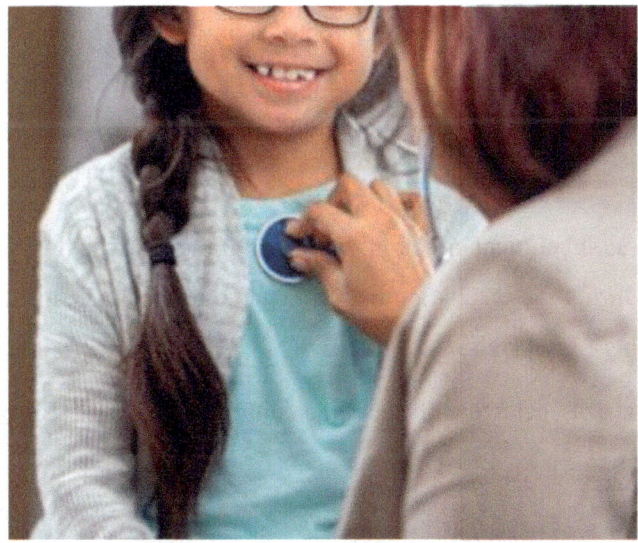

Clinicians now have more power to identify diseases thanks to advancements in technology.

Medical research has advanced significantly since the 1800s, enabling doctors to recognize symptoms with clarity. Today, a variety of tools are available to assist physicians in recognizing and evaluating symptoms that even patients might not have noticed.

These consist of:

- Stethoscope: This device allows a physician to listen to the heart and lungs.

- Spirometer: A tool for assessing lung function.
- Ophthalmoscope: This tool is used by eye specialists to look into the eye.
- X-ray imaging: This may reveal bone damage.
- Sphygmomanometer: This is a blood pressure measuring device that is worn around the arm.

Hundreds of new tools and methods for assessing indications were developed during the 20th century. Since physicians and patients no longer had to collaborate as closely to diagnose medical conditions, the terms "sign" and "symptom" acquired distinct meanings throughout this era of modern medical history.

Previously, doctors had to rely on patients to describe symptoms, but now they can see them. These are now categorized as signs, even though by the current criteria they would have been symptoms.

Symptoms

Three primary categories of symptoms exist:

- Symptoms that go away: Remitting symptoms occur when they become better or go away entirely. Common cold symptoms, for instance, can last for a few days before going away on their own without medical intervention.
- Prolonged or recurring symptoms are referred to as chronic symptoms. Chronic symptoms are frequently observed in long-term illnesses like cancer, diabetes, and asthma.
- Relapsing symptoms are those that have happened before, gone away, and then come again. For example, depressive symptoms may not manifest for years at a time, but they may reappear later.

Some illnesses don't have any symptoms at all. For instance, some tumors do not show symptoms until they are in their later, more aggressive stages, and a person may have high blood pressure for years without realizing it. These are referred to as asymptomatic conditions, and while the concept of symptoms is frequently associated with discomfort or aberrant function, asymptomatic illnesses can be fatal.

Many infections don't cause any symptoms. These are referred to as subclinical infections, and even if the individual who has them does not exhibit any symptoms, they can still spread. During the incubation period, when the infectious agent establishes itself in the body, the infection might still spread to other individuals.

The potential for problems unrelated to the illness itself is another risk associated with subclinical infections. For instance, preterm deliveries can result from untreated urinary tract infections (UTIs).

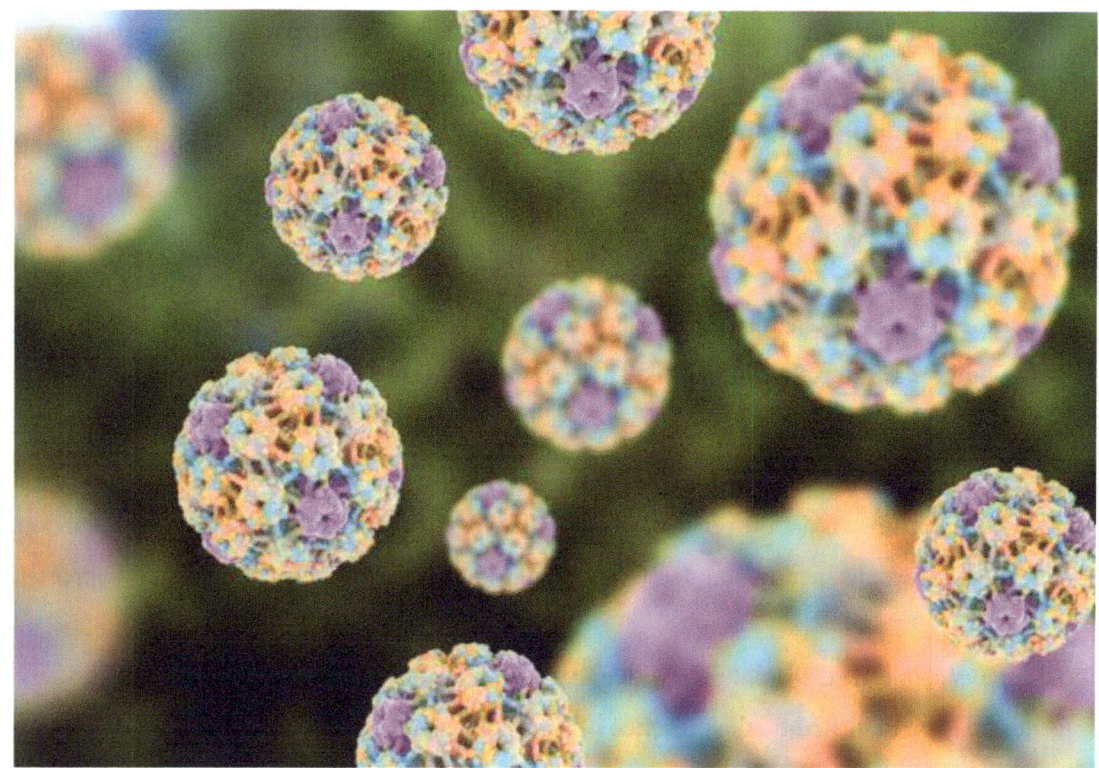

A lot of illnesses, including HPV, don't exhibit symptoms right away and can still spread to other people.

HIV, syphilis, hepatitis B and C, human papillomavirus (HPV), and herpes simplex virus (HSV) are a few examples of diseases that may not immediately produce symptoms.

Many people become aware of asymptomatic diseases for the first time when they visit a doctor, usually for a separate issue. In order to detect any hidden issues, it is crucial to get regular health examinations.

In their early stages, many malignancies show no symptoms. For instance, signs of prostate cancer do not appear until the disease has progressed to a particular stage. Since early cancer therapy is frequently essential, this is what makes some malignancies so hazardous.

Regular screening tests are crucial for at-risk persons because of this.

Signs

A medical sign is a physical reaction associated with a medical fact or feature that a doctor, nurse, or medical device notices when examining a patient. They may frequently be measured, and doing so can be crucial to determining the cause of a medical issue.

A patient may occasionally miss a sign because it doesn't seem important. In the hands of a medical practitioner who understands the relationship between this sign and the rest of the body, however, it may hold the secret to curing an underlying medical condition.

Here are a few instances of symptoms that a clinician may associate with an illness:

- High blood pressure: This may be a sign of an allergy, a pharmaceutical side effect, a cardiovascular issue, or a variety of other illnesses. To make a diagnosis, this is frequently paired with additional symptoms.
- Finger clumping: This could indicate a variety of hereditary illnesses or pulmonary conditions.

Physicians are trained to recognize symptoms that an untrained person might not consider significant.

The following categories apply to signs:

- Prognostic signs: These are indicators of what is ahead. They forecast the patient's outcome, including what will likely happen to them and how serious the condition is likely to be, rather than describing the nature of the illness.
- Anamnestic signs: These indicators indicate some aspects of a person's past health. Skin scars, for example, could be a sign of severe acne in the past.
- Diagnostic indicators: These indicators assist the physician in identifying a present medical issue. For instance, a male's elevated blood levels of prostate-specific antigen (PSA) could indicate prostate cancer or another prostate issue.
- Pathognomonic signs: A physician can be absolutely positive that a sign corresponds to a condition. For instance, a particular viral infection may be indicated by the presence of a particular microorganism in a blood sample.

Despite their distinctions, signals and symptoms are both ultimately ways the body expresses health issues and initiates the quest for a remedy.

It's crucial to pay attention to any symptoms you find on your own as well as any indicators a doctor may identify.

Clinical Presentation of First Aid: USMLE | Disease Diagnosis

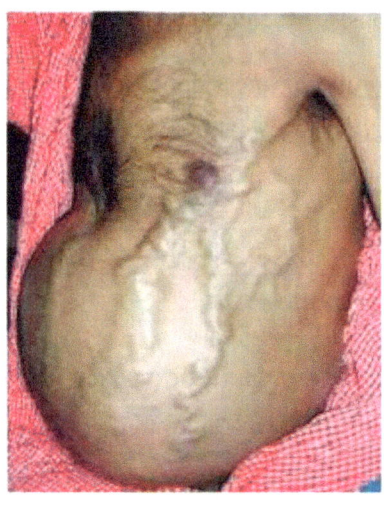

Budd-Chiari syndrome (posthepatic venous thrombosis)

Abdominal pain, ascites, hepatomegaly

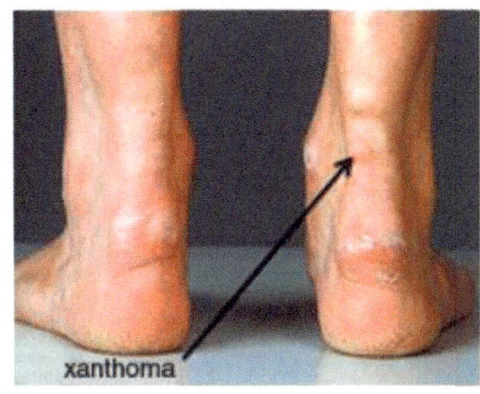

Achilles tendon xanthoma

Familial hypercholesterolemia (Decreased LDL receptor signaling)

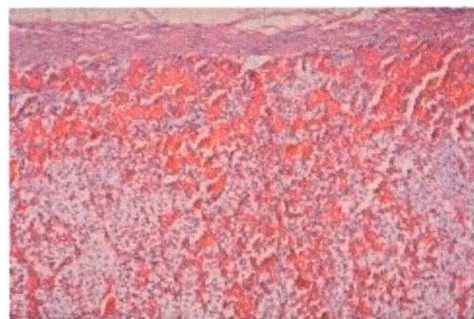

Adrenal hemorrhage, hypotension, DIC

Waterhouse-Friderichsen syndrome (meningococcemia)

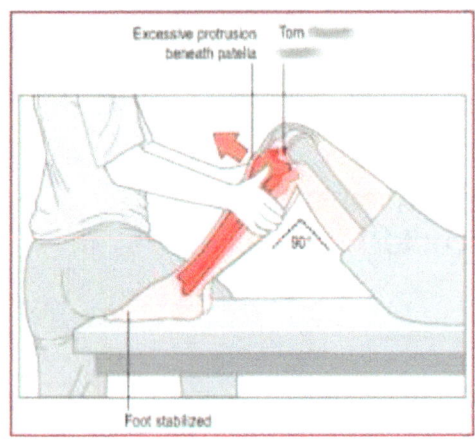

Anterior "drawer sign" + — Anterior cruciate ligament injury

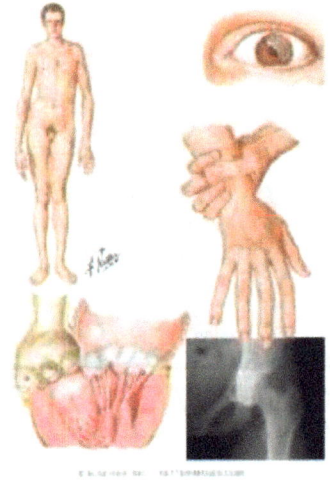

Arachnodactyly, lens dislocation, aortic dissection, hyperflexible joints — Marfan syndrome (fibrillin defect)

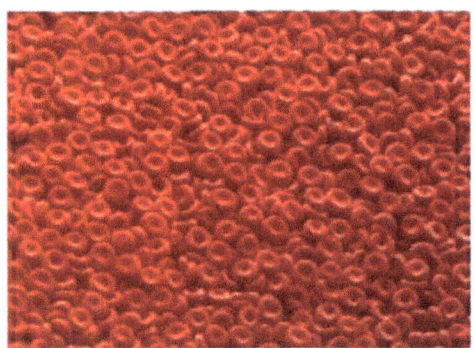

Athlete with polycythemia — 2° to erythropoietin injection

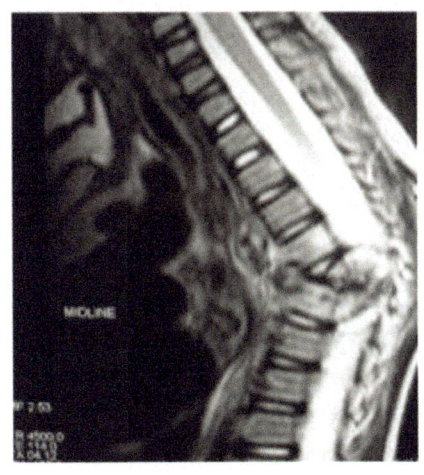

Back pain, fever, night sweats, weight loss

Pott disease (vertebral TB)

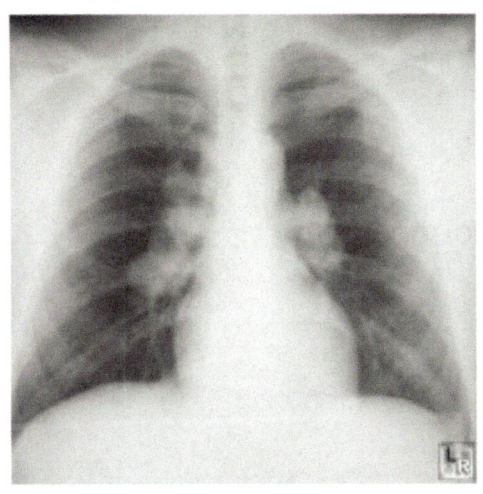

Bilateral hilar adenopathy, uveitis

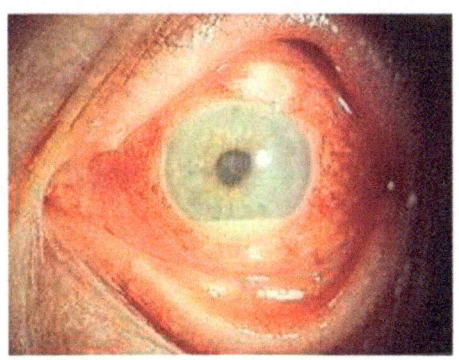

Sarcoidosis (noncaseating granulomas)

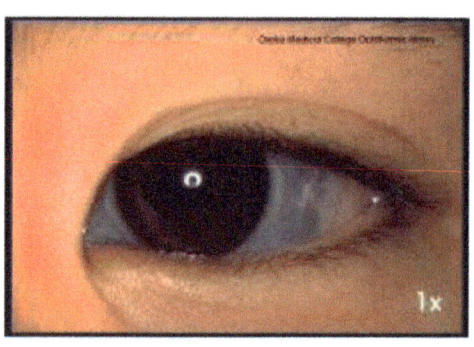

Blue sclera

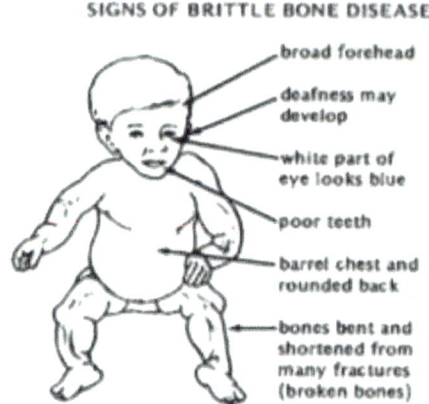

Osteogenesis imperfecta (type I collagen defect)

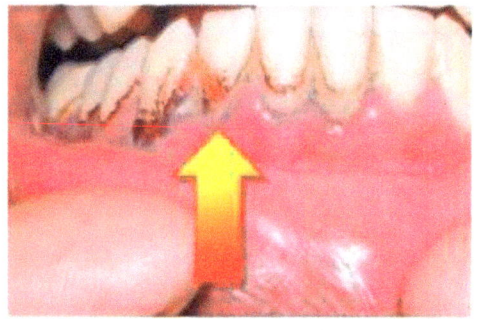

Bluish line on gingiva

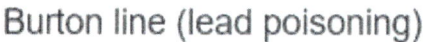

Burton line (lead poisoning)

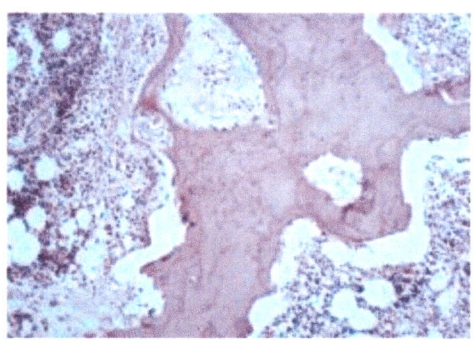

Bone pain, bone enlargement, arthritis

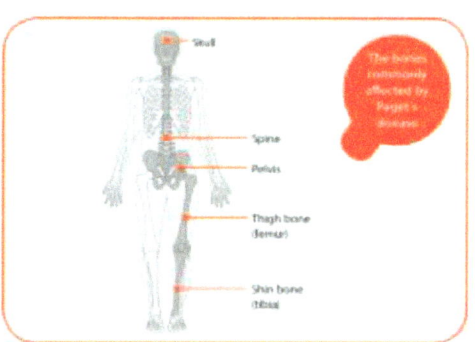

Paget disease of bone (Increased osteoblastic and osteoclastic activity)

Bounding pulses (strong & forceful), diastolic heart murmur, head bobbing

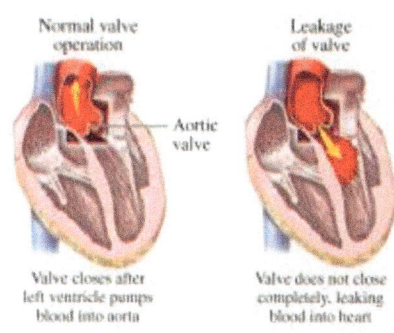

Aortic regurgitation

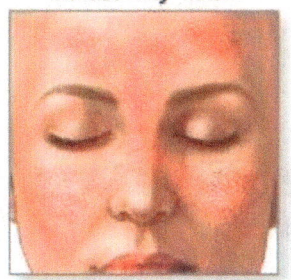

"Butterfly" facial rash and Raynaud phenomenon in a young female

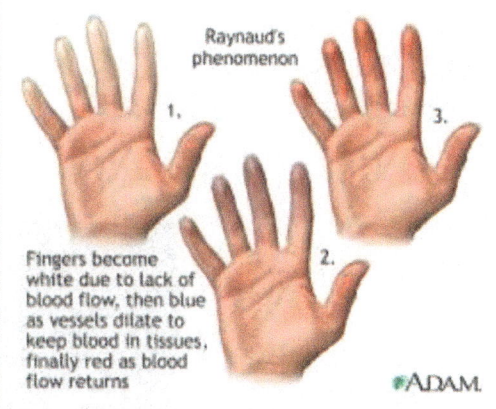

Systemic lupus erythematosus

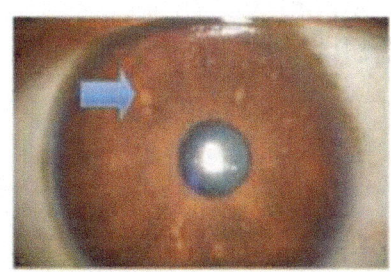

Café-au-lait spots, Lisch nodules (iris hamartoma)

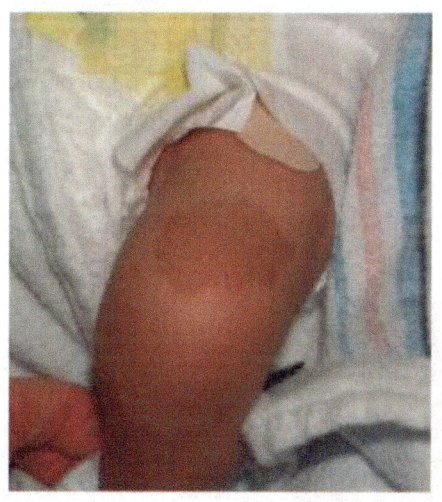

Neurofibromatosis type I (+ pheochromocytoma, optic gliomas)

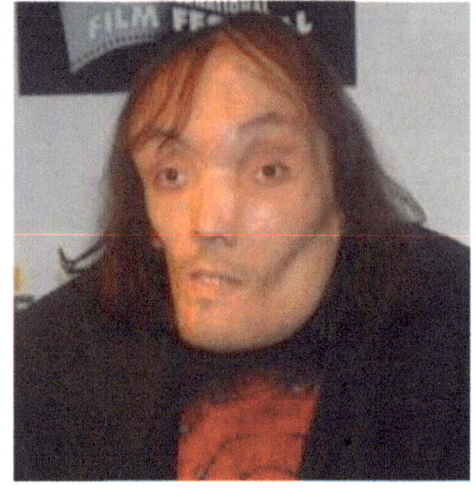

Café-au-lait spots, polyostotic fibrous dysplasia, precocious

McCune-Albright syndrome (mosaic G-protein signaling mutation)

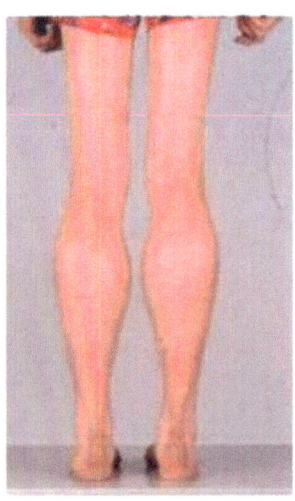

Calf pseudohypertrophy

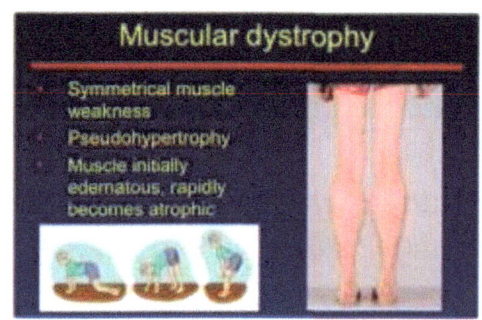

Muscular dystrophy (most commonly Duchenne): X-linked recessive deletion of dystrophin gene

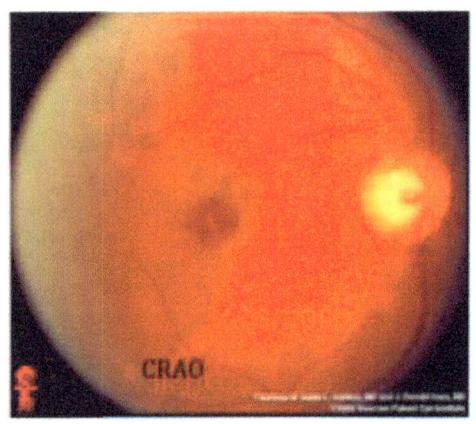

"Cherry-red spots" on macula

Tay-Sachs (ganglioside accumulation) or Niemann-Pick (sphingomyelin accumulation), central retinal artery occlusion

Chest pain on exertion

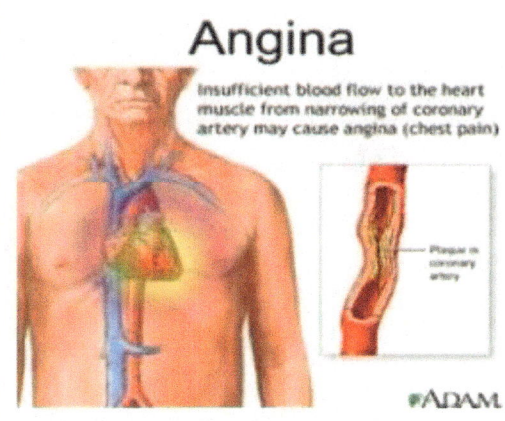

Angina (stable: with moderate exertion; unstable: with minimal exertion)

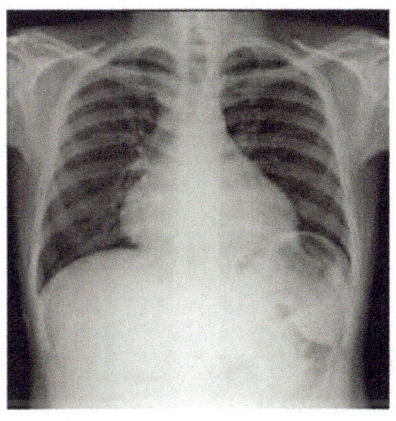

Chest pain, pericardial effusion/friction rub, persistent fever following MI

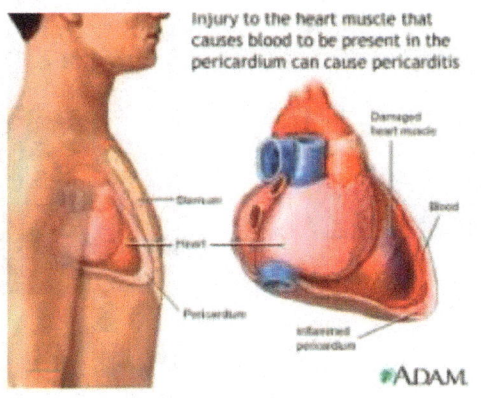

Dressler syndrome (autoimmune-mediated post-MI fibrinous pericarditis, 1–12 weeks after acute episode)

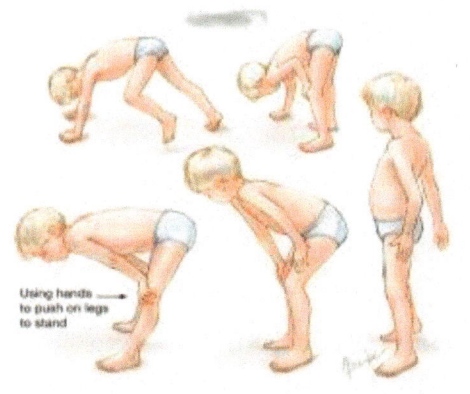

Child uses arms to stand up from squat

Gowers sign (Duchenne muscular dystrophy)

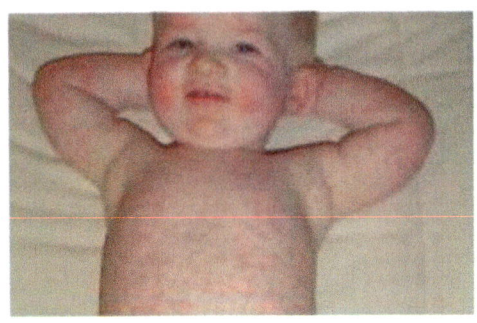

Child with fever later develops red rash on face that spreads to body

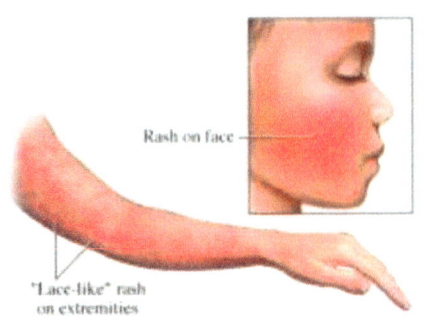

"Slapped cheeks" (erythema infectiosum/fifth disease: parvovirus B19)

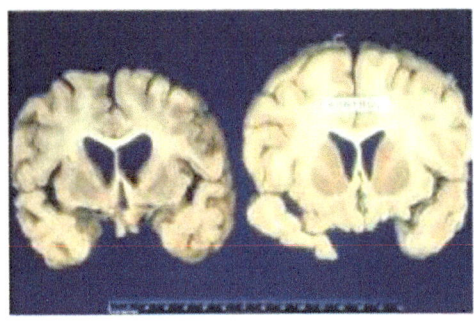

Chorea, dementia, caudate degeneration

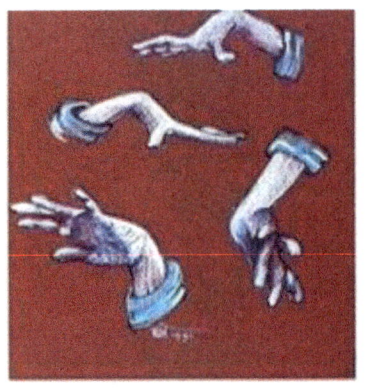

Huntington disease (autosomal dominant CAG repeat expansion)

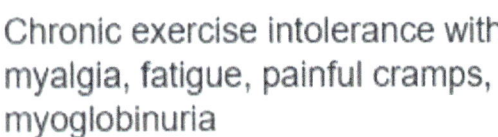

Chronic exercise intolerance with myalgia, fatigue, painful cramps, myoglobinuria

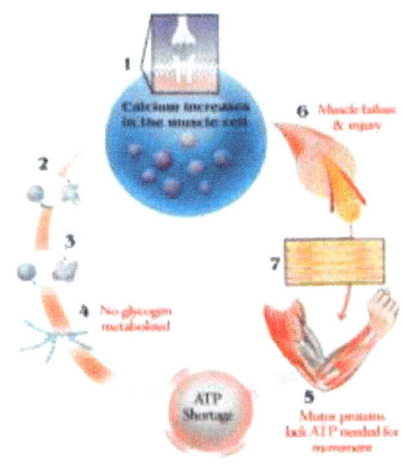

McArdle disease (muscle glycogen phosphorylase deficiency)

Cold intolerance

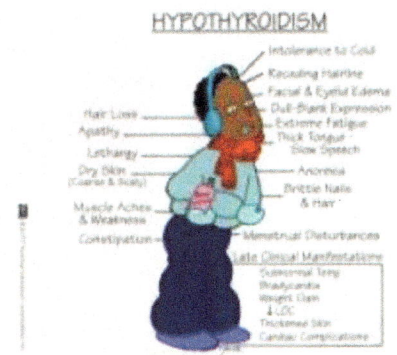

Hypothyroidism

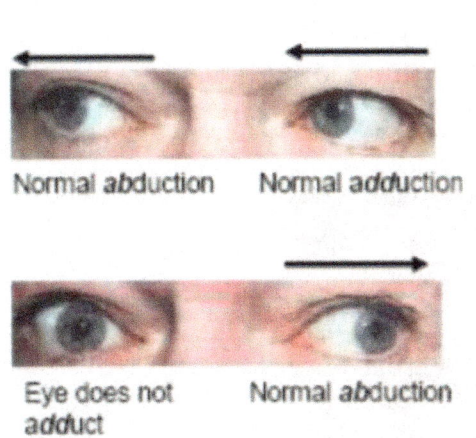

Conjugate lateral gaze palsy, horizontal diplopia

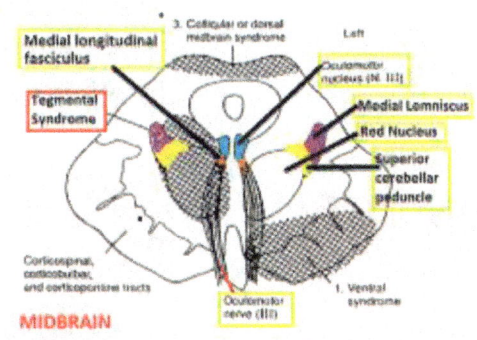

Internuclear ophthalmoplegia (damage to medial longitudinal fasciculus; bilateral [multiple sclerosis], unilateral [stroke])

Continuous "machine-like" heart murmur

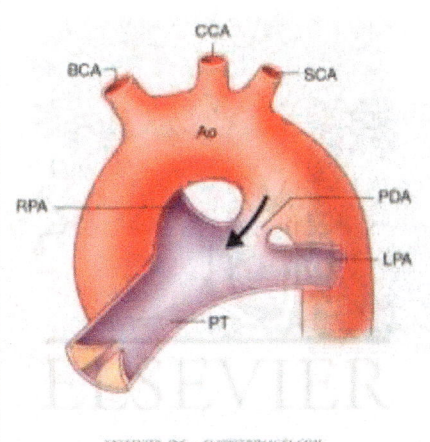

PDA (close with indomethacin; open or maintain with misoprostol)

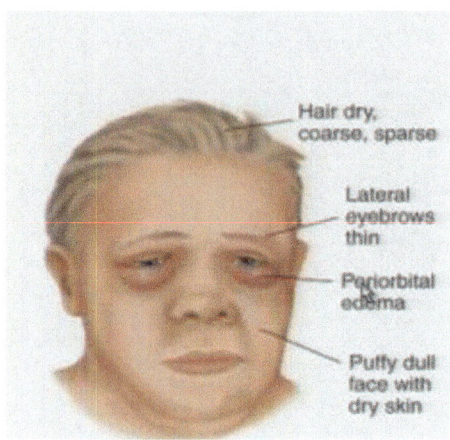

Cutaneous/dermal edema due to connective tissue deposition

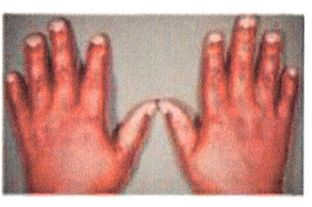
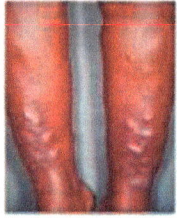

Myxedema (caused by hypothyroidism, Graves disease [pretibial myxedema])

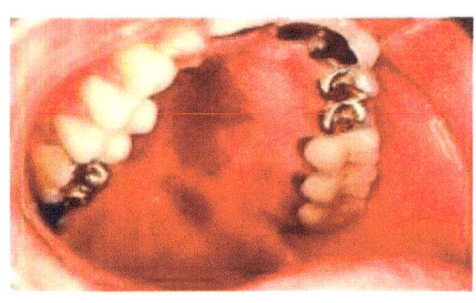

Dark purple skin/mouth nodules in a patient with AIDS

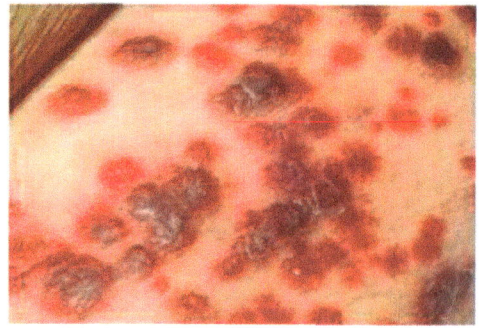

Kaposi sarcoma, associated with HHV-8

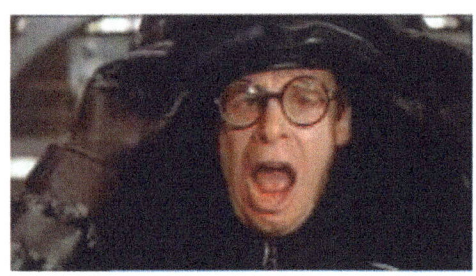

Deep, labored breathing/hyperventilation

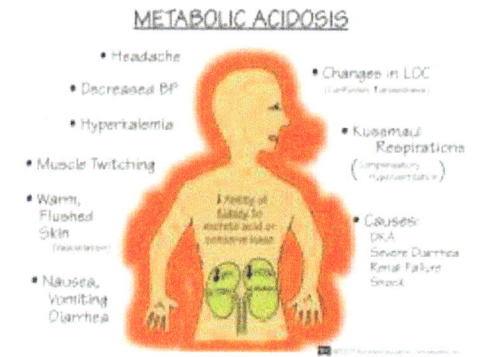

Kussmaul respirations (diabetic ketoacidosis)

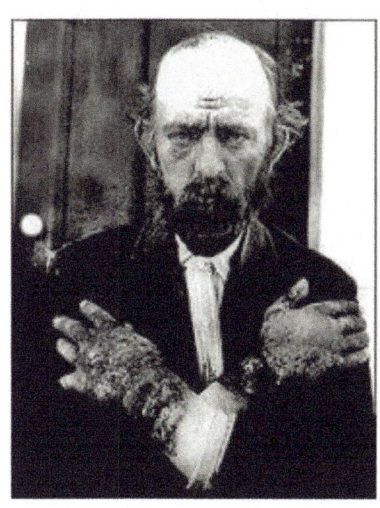

Dermatitis, dementia, diarrhea

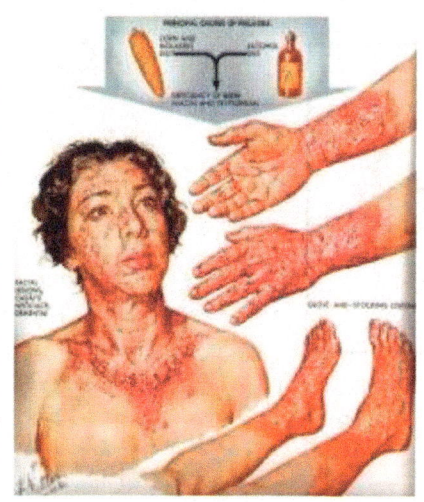

Pellagra (niacin [vitamin B3] deficiency)

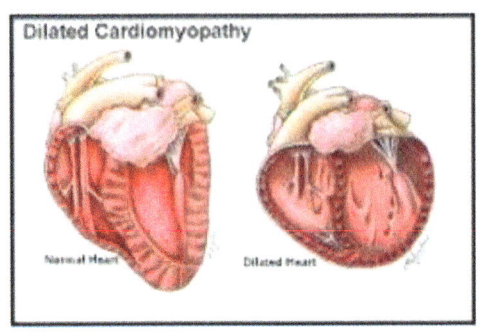

Dilated cardiomyopathy, edema, alcoholism or malnutrition

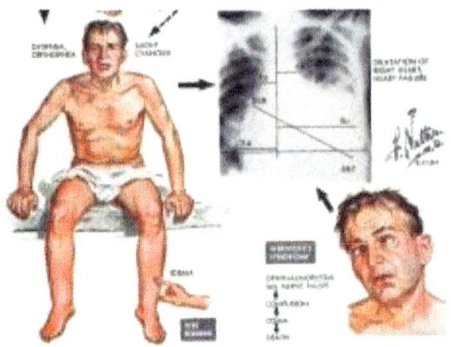

Wet beriberi (thiamine [vitamin B1] deficiency)

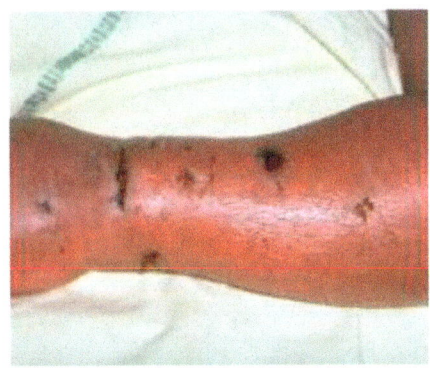

Dog or cat bite resulting in infection

Pasteurella multocida (cellulitis at inoculation site)

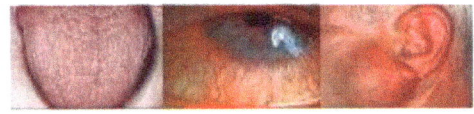

Dry eyes, dry mouth, arthritis

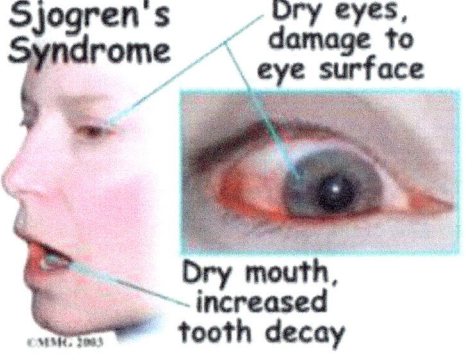

Sjögren syndrome (autoimmune destruction of exocrine glands)

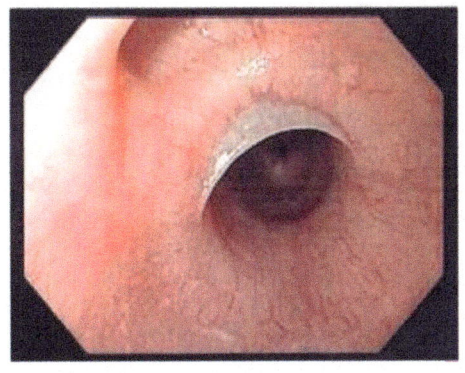

Dysphagia (esophageal webs), glossitis, iron deficiency anemia

Plummer-Vinson syndrome (may progress to esophageal squamous cell carcinoma)

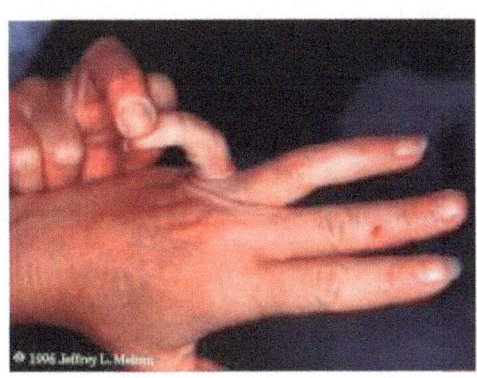

Elastic skin, hypermobility of joints

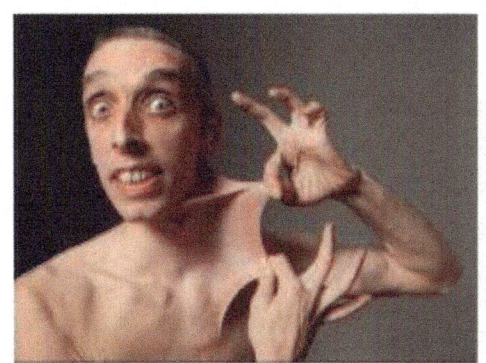

Ehlers-Danlos syndrome (type III collagen defect)

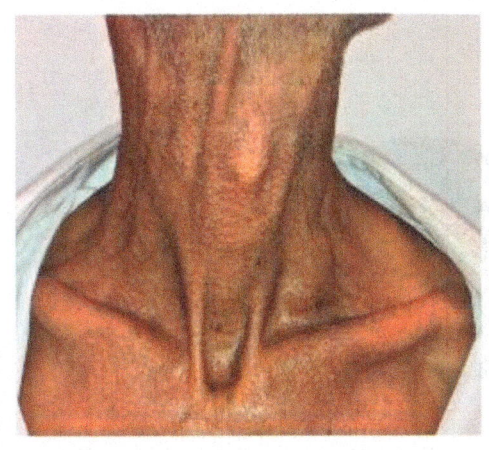

Enlarged, hard left supraclavicular node

Virchow node (abdominal metastasis)

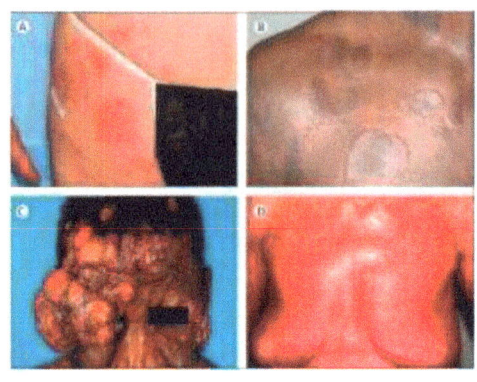

Erythroderma, lymphadenopathy, hepatosplenomegaly, atypical T cells

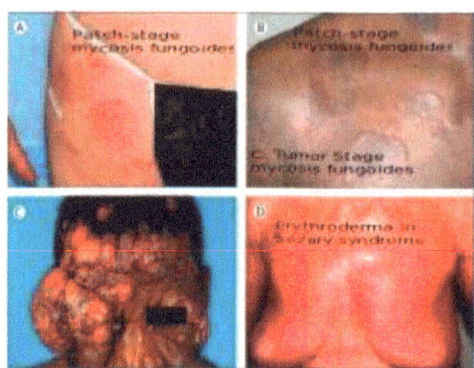

Mycosis fungoides (cutaneous T-cell lymphoma) or Sézary syndrome (mycosis fungoides + malignant T cells in blood)

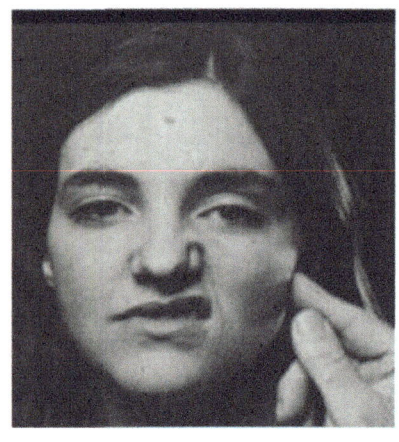

Facial muscle spasm upon tapping

Chvostek sign (hypocalcemia)

Fat, female, forty, and fertile

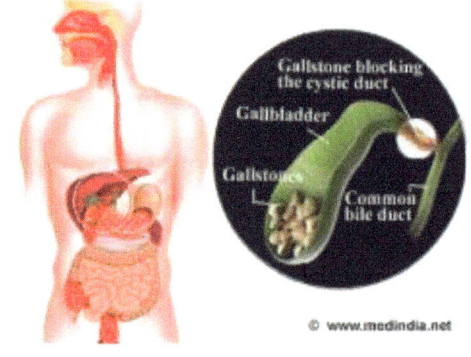

Cholelithiasis (gallstones)

Fever, chills, headache, myalgia following antibiotic treatment for syphilis

Jarisch-Herxheimer reaction (rapid lysis of spirochetes results in toxin release)

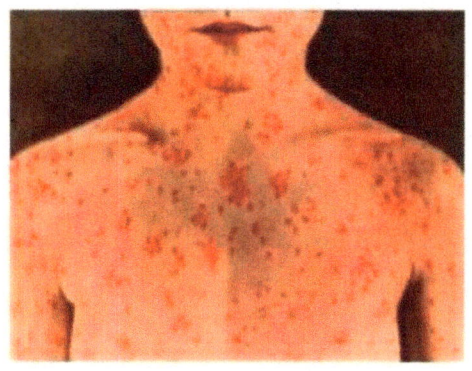 Fever, cough, conjunctivitis, coryza, diffuse rash, Koplik spots (Buccal Mucosa)	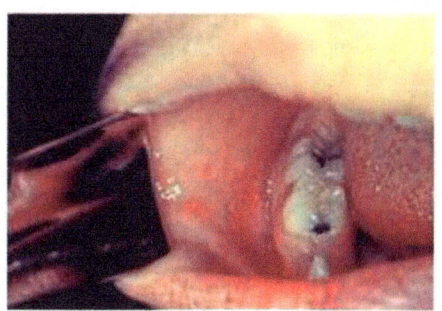 Measles
Fever, night sweats, weight loss	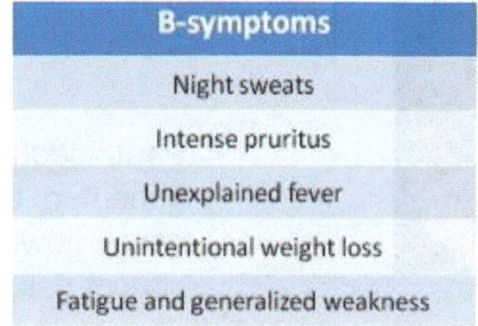 B symptoms (staging) of lymphoma
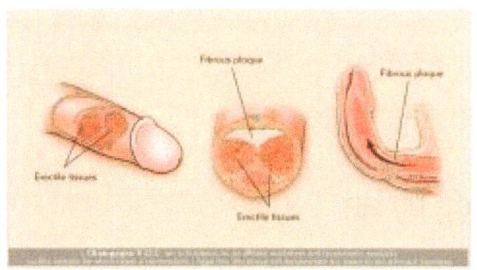 Fibrous plaques in soft tissue of penis	Peyronie disease (connective tissue disorder)
Gout, intellectual disability, self-mutilating behavior in a boy	Lesch-Nyhan syndrome (HGPRT deficiency, X-linked recessive)

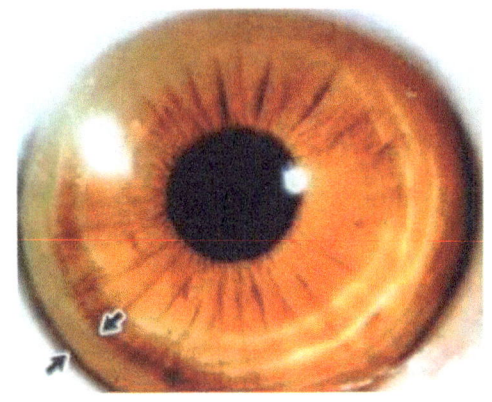 Green-yellow rings around peripheral cornea	Kayser-Fleischer rings (copper accumulation from Wilson disease)
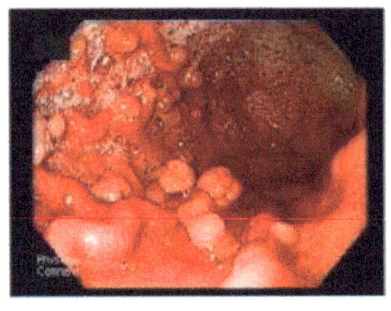 Hamartomatous GI polyps, hyperpigmentation of mouth/feet/hands	Peutz-Jeghers syndrome (inherited, benign polyposis can cause bowel obstruction; Increased cancer risk, mainly GI)
Hepatosplenomegaly, osteoporosis, neurologic symptoms	Gaucher disease (glucocerebrosidase deficiency -> lysosomal storage disease characterized by an accumulation of glucocerebrosides.)
Hereditary nephritis, sensorineural hearing loss, cataracts	Alport syndrome (mutation in collagen IV)

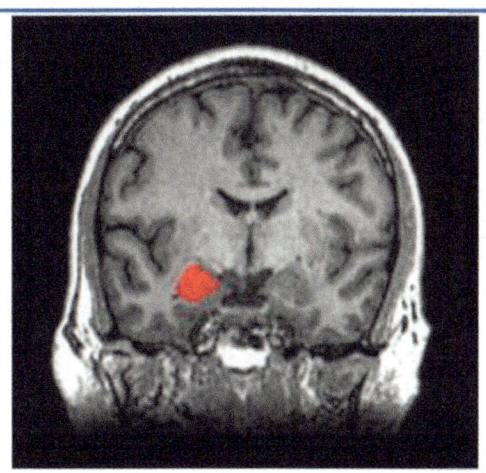 Hyperphagia, hypersexuality, hyperorality, hyperdocility	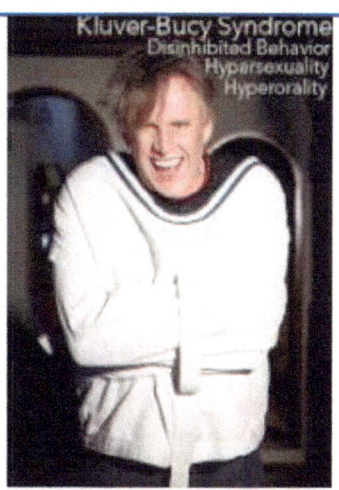 Klüver-Bucy syndrome (bilateral amygdala lesion)
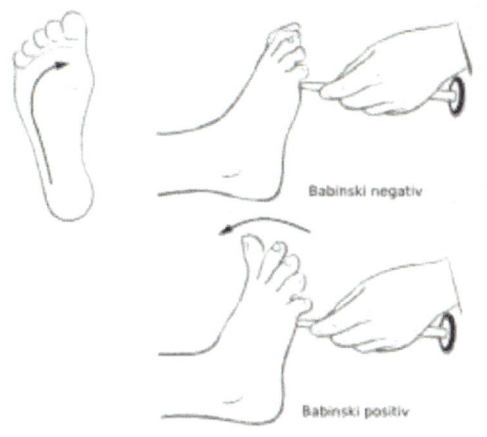 Hyperreflexia, hypertonia, Babinski sign present	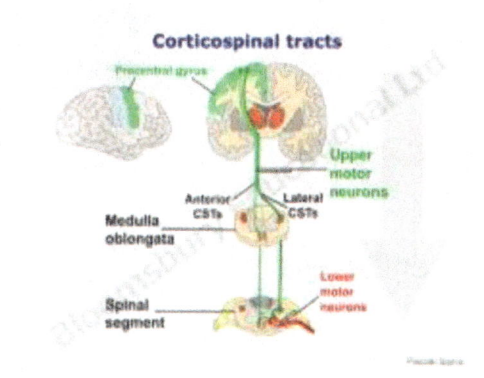 UMN damage
Hyporeflexia, hypotonia, atrophy, fasciculations (small, local, involuntary twitch)	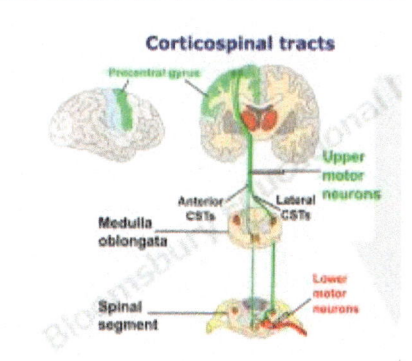 LMN damage

Hypoxemia, polycythemia, hypercapnia (high CO2)

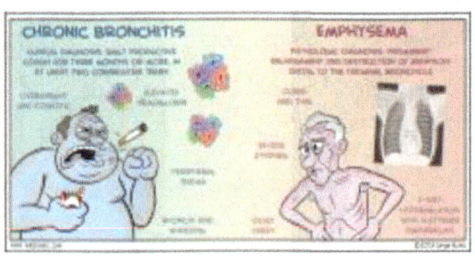

"Blue bloater" (chronic bronchitis: hyperplasia of mucous cells)

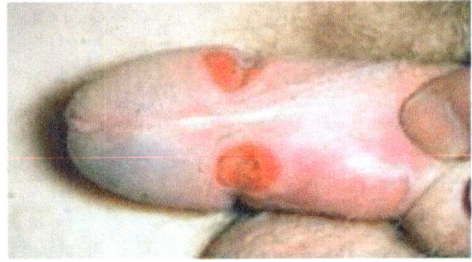

Indurated, ulcerated genital lesion

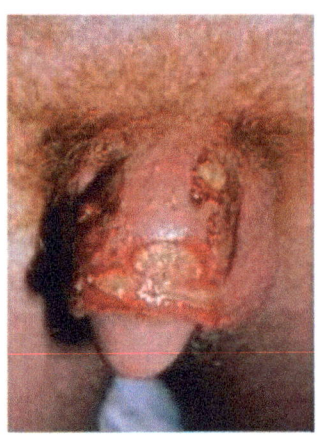

SIDE 1: Nonpainful chancre (1° syphilis, Treponema pallidum)

SIDE 2: Painful chancroid with exudate (Haemophilus ducreyi)

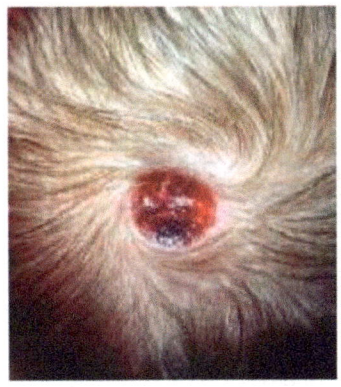 Infant with cleft lip/palate, microcephaly or holoprosencephaly, polydactyly, cutis aplasia	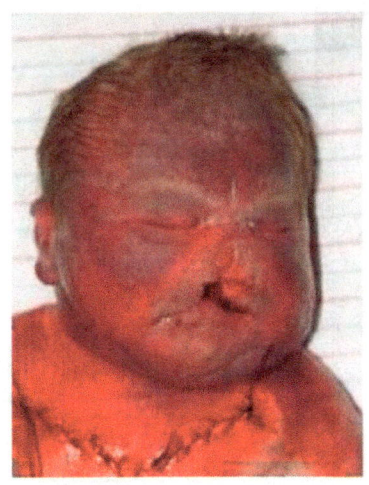 Patau syndrome (trisomy 13)
Infant with failure to thrive, hepatosplenomegaly, and neurodegeneration	Niemann-Pick disease (genetic sphingomyelinase deficiency)
Infant with hypoglycemia, failure to thrive, and hepatomegaly	Cori disease (debranching enzyme deficiency) or Von Gierke disease (glucose-6-phosphatase deficiency, more severe)
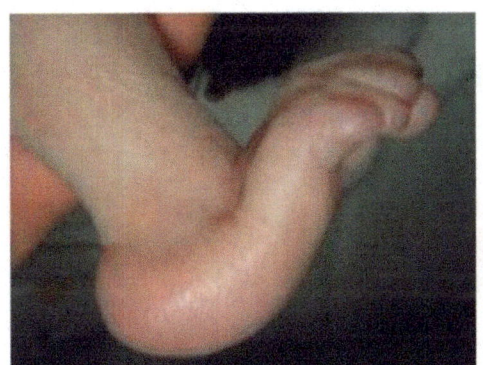 Infant with microcephaly, rocker-bottom feet, clenched hands, and structural heart defect	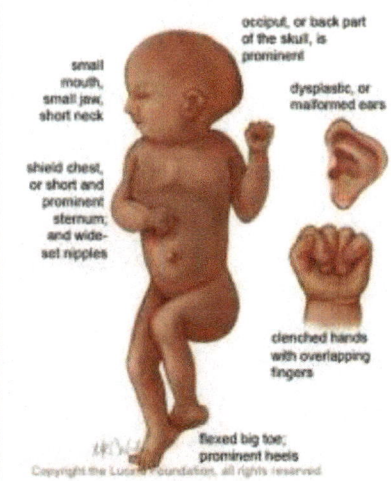 Edwards syndrome (trisomy 18)
Jaundice, palpable distended non-tender gallbladder	Courvoisier sign (distal obstruction of biliary tree)

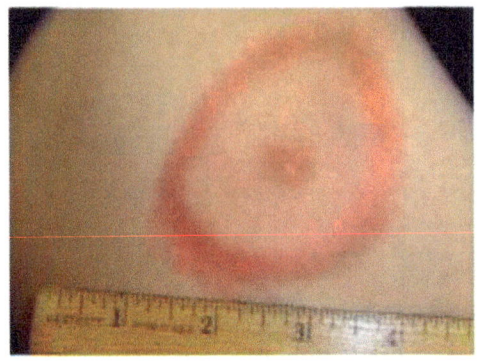 Large rash with bull's-eye appearance	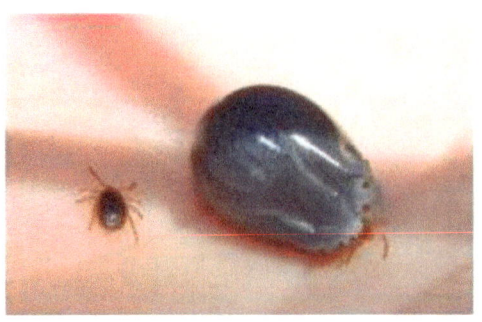 Erythema chronicum migrans from Ixodes tick bite (Lyme disease: Borrelia)
Lucid interval after traumatic brain injury	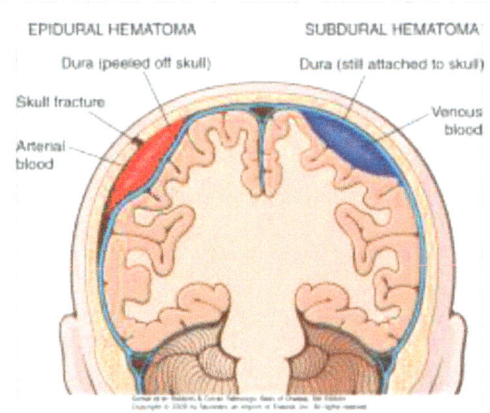 Epidural hematoma (middle meningeal artery rupture)
Male child, recurrent infections, no mature B cells	Bruton disease (X-linked agammaglobulinemia)
Mucosal bleeding and prolonged bleeding time	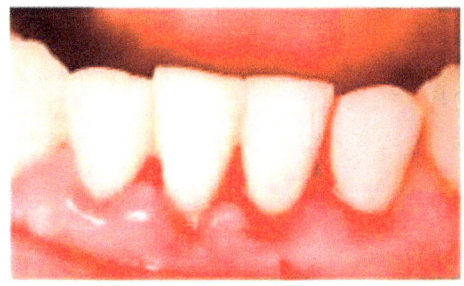 Glanzmann thrombasthenia (defect in platelet aggregation due to lack of GpIIb/IIIa)

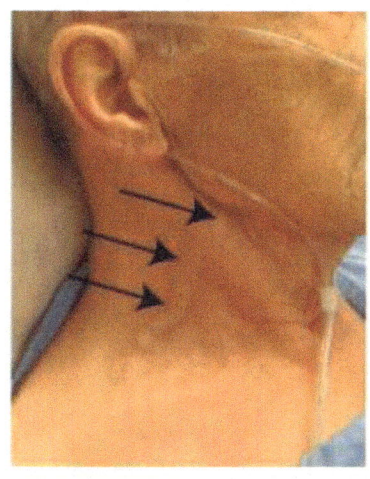

Muffled heart sounds, distended neck veins, hypotension

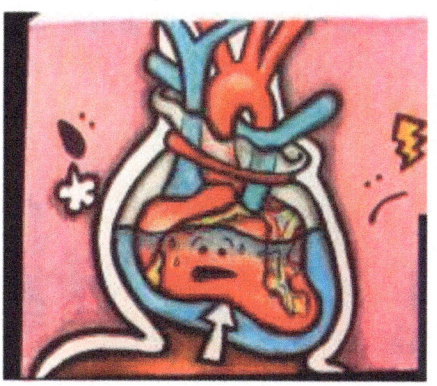

Beck triad of cardiac tamponade

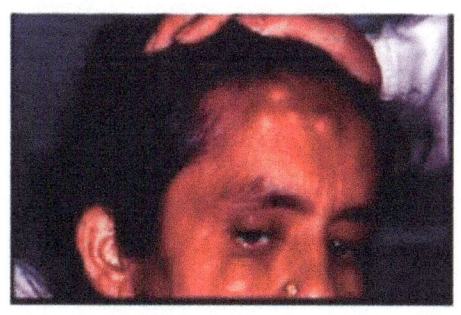

Multiple colon polyps, osteomas/soft tissue tumors, impacted/ supernumerary teeth

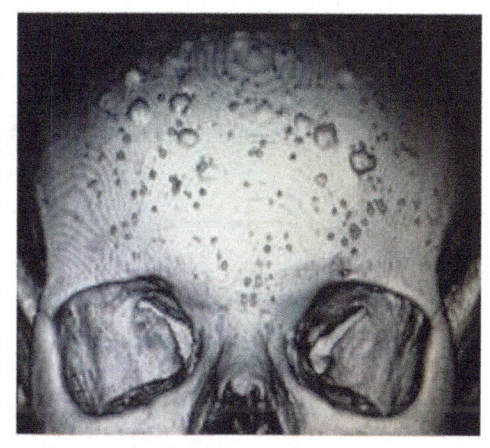

Gardner syndrome (subtype of FAP)

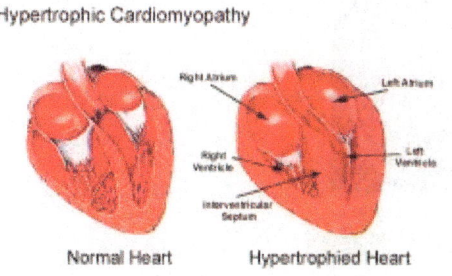

Myopathy (infantile hypertrophic cardiomyopathy), exercise intolerance

Pompe disease (lysosomal α-1,4-glucosidase deficiency)

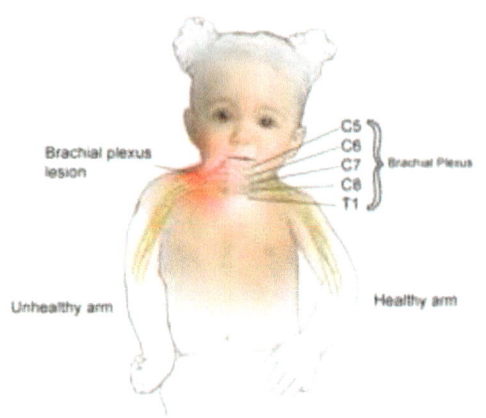

Neonate with arm paralysis following difficult birth

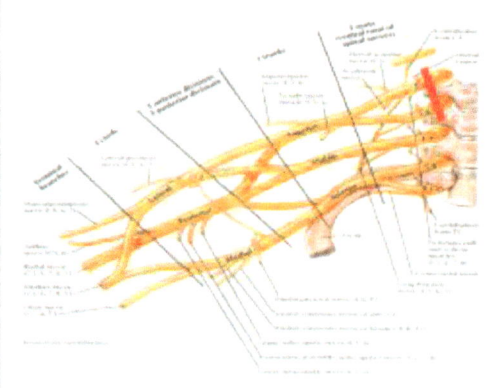

Erb-Duchenne palsy (superior trunk [C5–C6] brachial plexus injury: "waiter's tip")

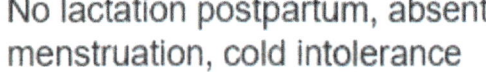

No lactation postpartum, absent menstruation, cold intolerance

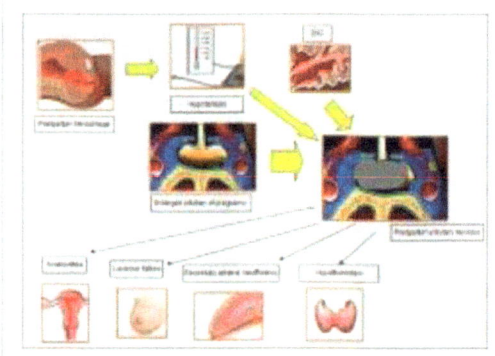

Sheehan syndrome (pituitary infarction)

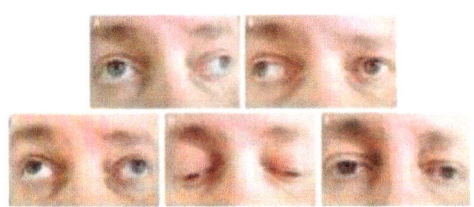

Nystagmus, intention tremor, scanning speech, bilateral internuclear ophthalmoplegia

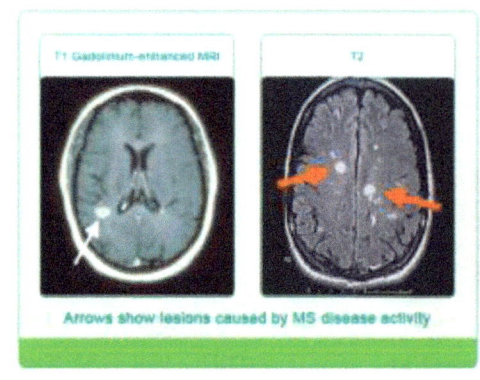

Multiple sclerosis

Oscillating slow/fast breathing	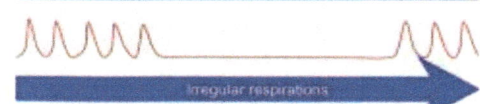 Cheyne-Stokes respirations (central apnea in CHF or increased intracranial pressure)
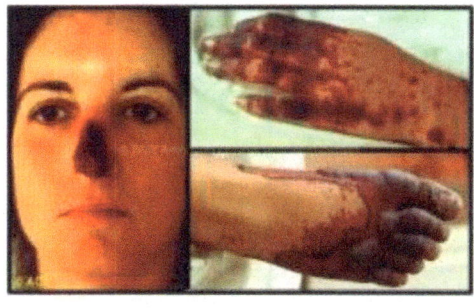 Painful blue fingers/toes, hemolytic anemia	Cold agglutinin disease (autoimmune hemolytic anemia caused by Mycoplasma pneumoniae, infectious mononucleosis)
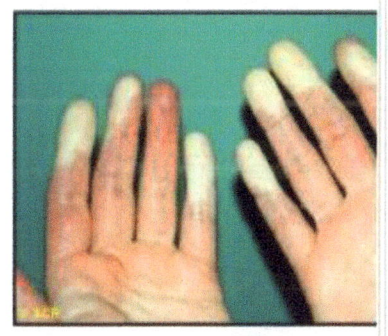 Painful, pale, cold fingers/toes	Raynaud phenomenon (vasospasm in extremities, response to cold or emotional stress, can be 2° to connective tissue disease, SLE, or CREST)
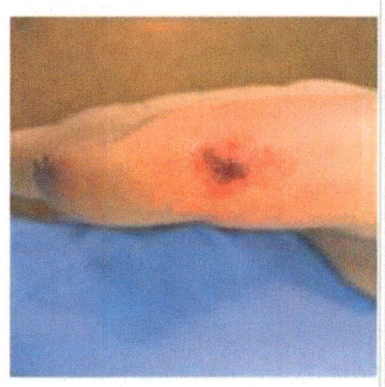	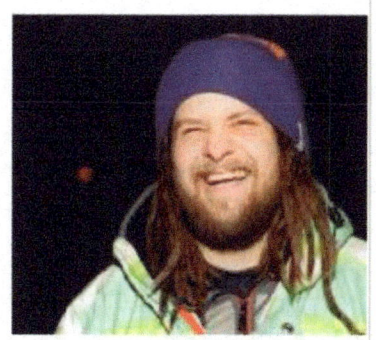

Painful, raised red lesions on pad of fingers/toes 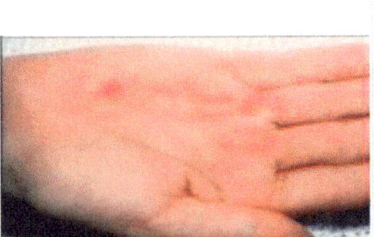 Painless erythematous lesions on palms and soles	Osler nodes (infective endocarditis, immune complex deposition) 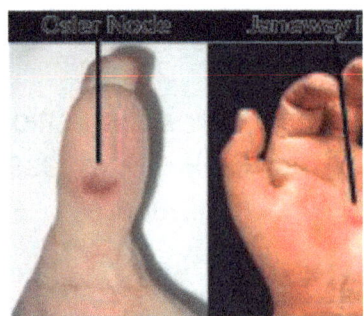 Janeway lesions (infective endocarditis, septic emboli/ microabscesses)
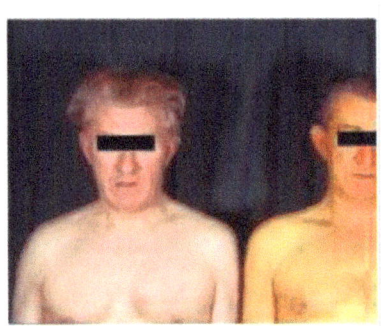 Painless jaundice	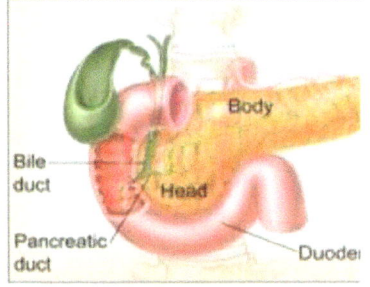 Cancer of the pancreatic head obstructing bile duct

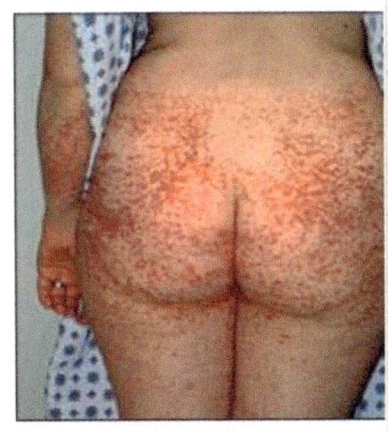

Henoch-Schönlein purpura (IgA vasculitis affecting skin and kidneys)

Palpable purport (small hemorrhages) on buttocks/legs, joint pain, abdominal pain (child), hematuria (kidney involvement)

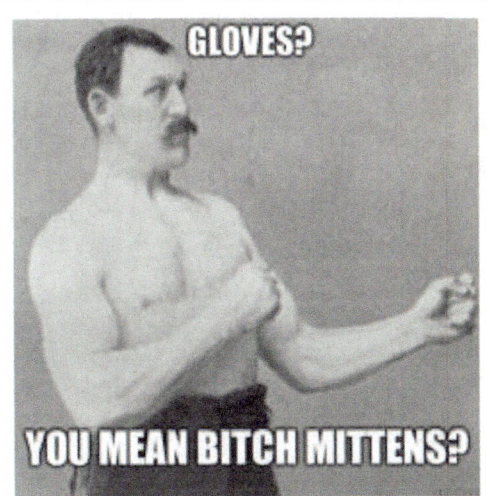

Pancreatic, pituitary, parathyroid tumors

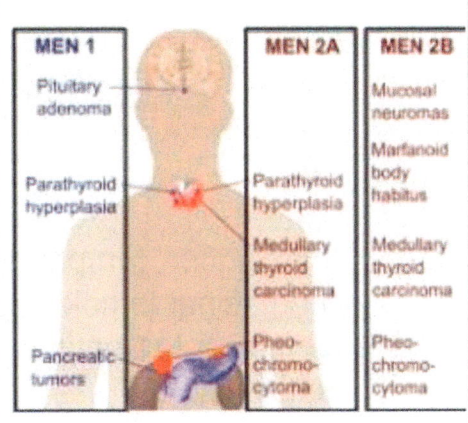

MEN 1 (autosomal dominant)

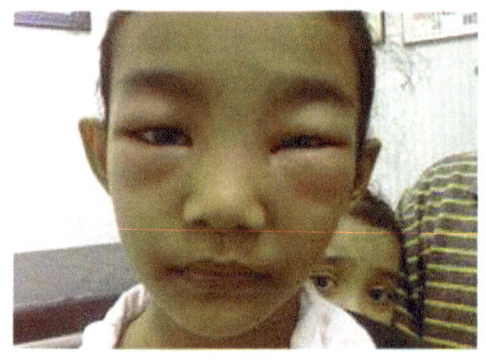

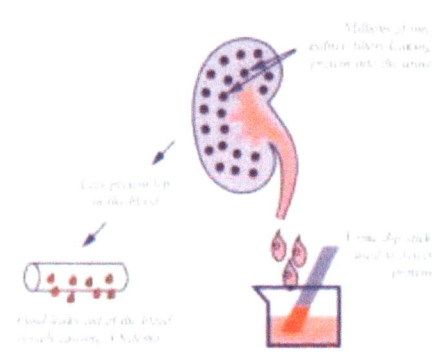

Periorbital and/or peripheral edema, proteinuria, hypoalbuminemia, hypercholesterolemia

Nephrotic syndrome

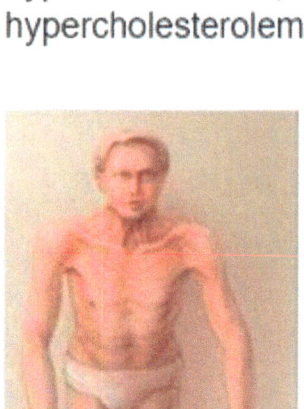

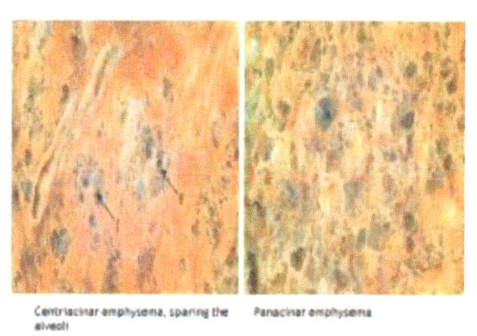

Centriacinar emphysema, sparing the alveoli   Panacinar emphysema

Pink complexion, dyspnea, hyperventilation

"Pink puffer" (emphysema: centriacinar [smoking], panacinar [α1-antitrypsin deficiency])

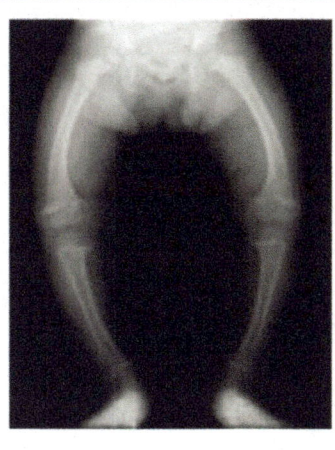

Polyuria, renal tubular acidosis type II, growth failure, electrolyte imbalances, hypophosphatemic rickets

Fanconi syndrome (proximal tubular reabsorption defect)

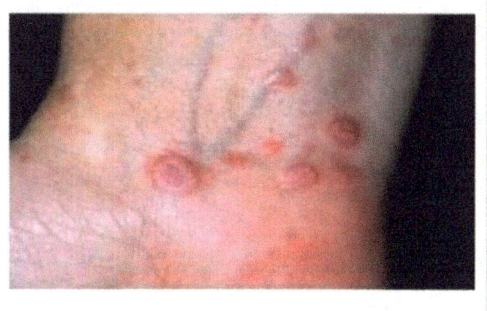

Pruritic, purple, polygonal planar papules and plaques (6 P's)

Lichen planus

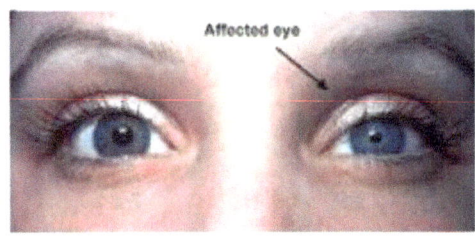 Ptosis, miosis, anhidrosis	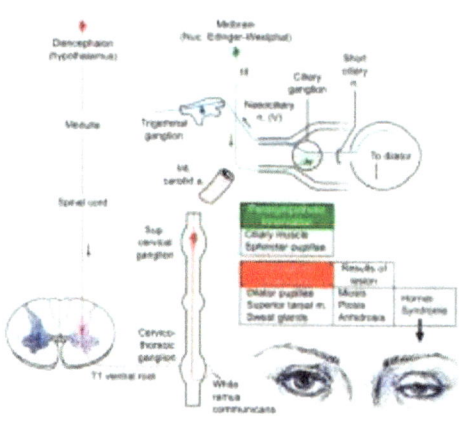 Horner syndrome (sympathetic chain lesion)
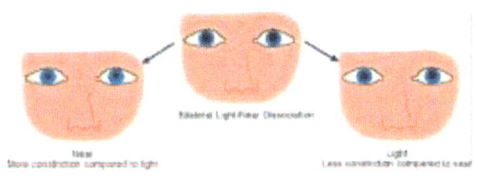 Pupil accommodates but doesn't react	Argyll Robertson pupil (neurosyphilis)
Rapidly progressive leg weakness that ascends following GI/ upper respiratory infection	Guillain-Barré syndrome (acute autoimmune inflammatory demyelinating polyneuropathy)
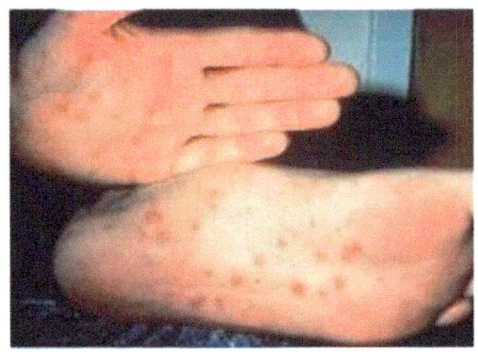 Rash on palms and soles	Coxsackie A, 2° syphilis, Rocky Mountain spotted fever
Recurrent colds, unusual eczema, high serum IgE	Hyper-IgE syndrome (Job syndrome: neutrophil chemotaxis abnormality)

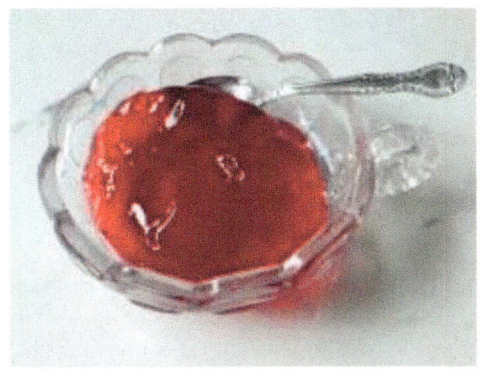

Red "currant jelly" sputum in alcoholic or diabetic patients

Klebsiella pneumoniae

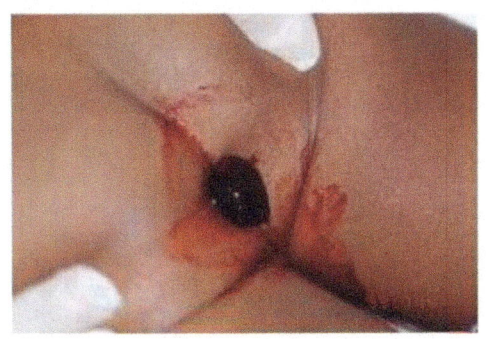

Red "currant jelly" stools

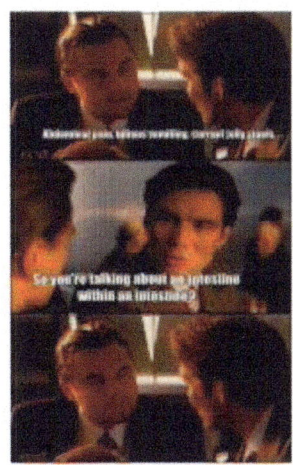

Acute mesenteric ischemia (adults), intussusception (infants, telescoping of the intestine)

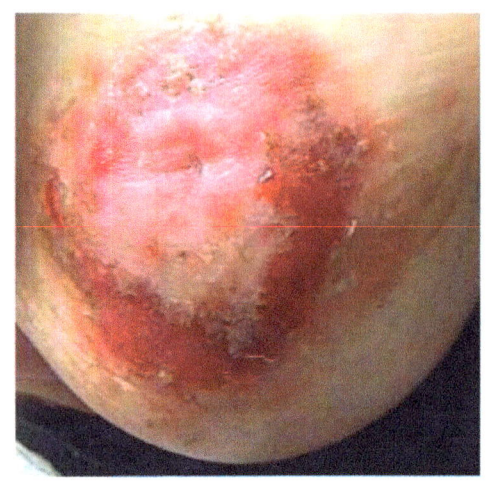 Red, itchy, swollen rash of nipple/areola	Paget disease of the breast (sign of underlying neoplasm)
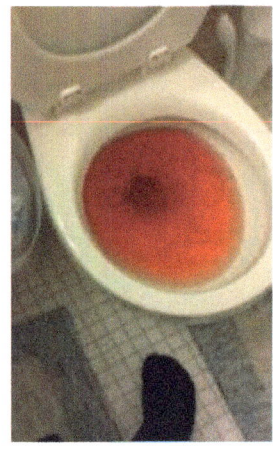 Red urine in the morning, fragile RBCs	Paroxysmal nocturnal hemoglobinuria
Renal cell carcinoma (bilateral), hemangioblastomas, angiomatosis, pheochromocytoma	von Hippel-Lindau disease (dominant tumor suppressor gene mutation)
Resting tremor, rigidity, akinesia, postural instability	Parkinson disease (nigrostriatal dopamine depletion)

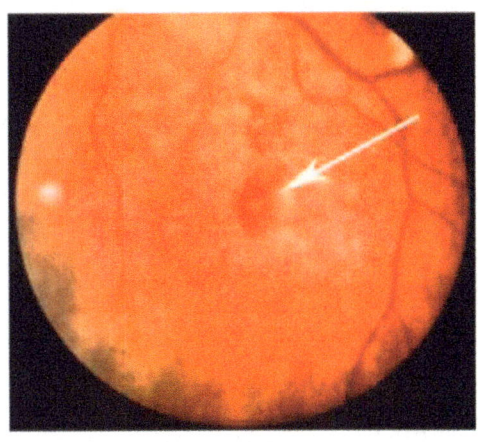

Retinal hemorrhages with pale centers

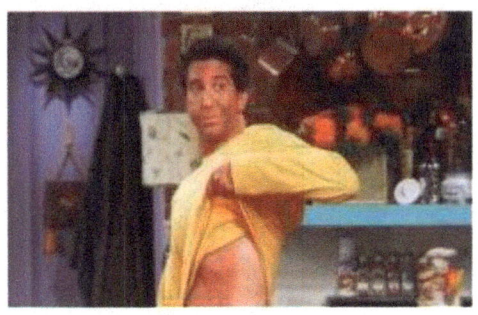

Roth spots (bacterial endocarditis)

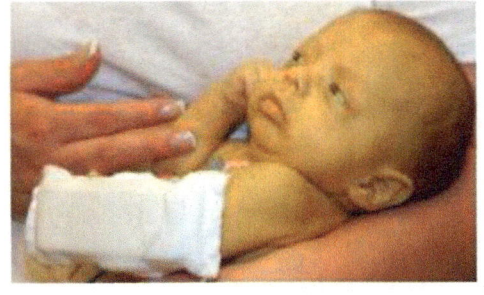

Severe jaundice in neonate

Crigler-Najjar syndrome (congenital unconjugated hyperbilirubinemia)

Severe RLQ pain with palpation of LLQ

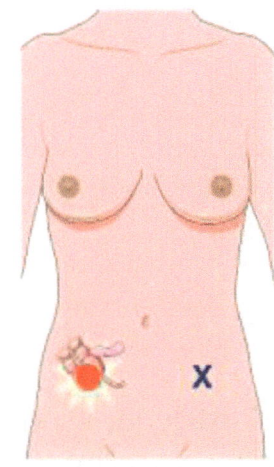

Rovsing sign (acute appendicitis)

Severe RLQ pain with rebound tenderness

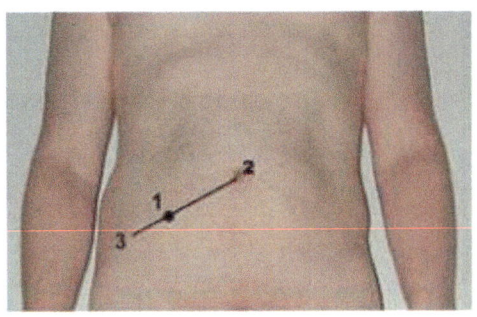

McBurney sign (McBurney's point (1), located two thirds the distance from the umbilicus (2) to the rightanterior superior iliac spine (3),acute appendicitis)

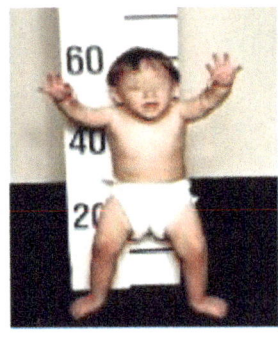

Short stature, increased incidence of tumors/leukemia, aplastic anemia

Fanconi anemia (genetic loss of DNA crosslink repair; often progresses to AML)

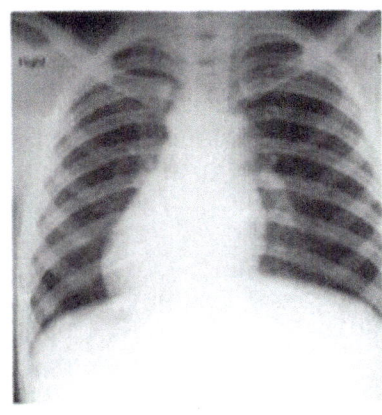

Situs inversus, chronic sinusitis, bronchiectasis, infertility

Kartagener syndrome (dynein arm defect affecting cilia)

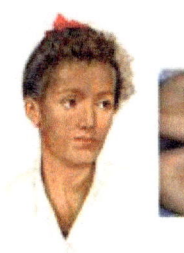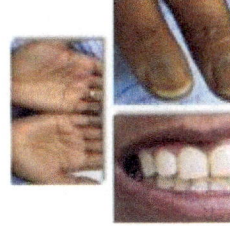 Skin hyperpigmentation, hypotension, fatigue	Addison disease (1° adrenocortical insufficiency causes high ACTH and high α-MSH production)
Slow, progressive muscle weakness in boys	Becker muscular dystrophy (X-linked missense mutation in dystrophin; less severe than Duchenne)
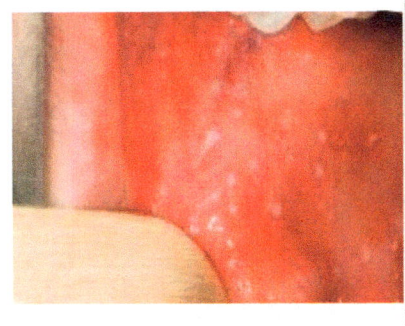 Small, irregular red spots on buccal/lingual mucosa with blue-white centers	Koplik spots (measles; rubeola virus)

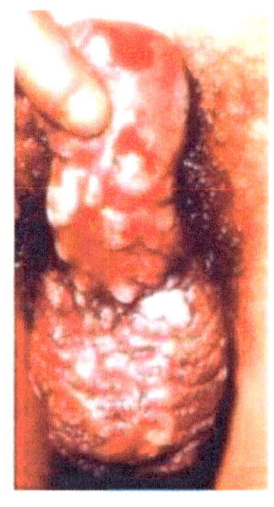

Condylomata lata (2° syphilis)

Smooth, flat, moist, painless white lesions on genitals

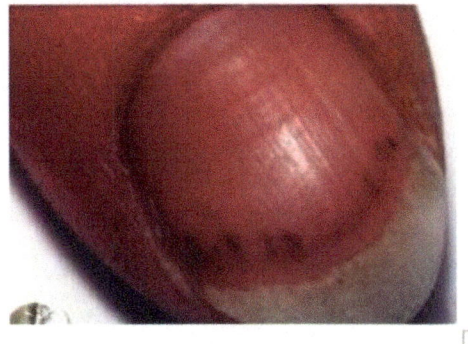 Splinter hemorrhages in fingernails	Bacterial endocarditis
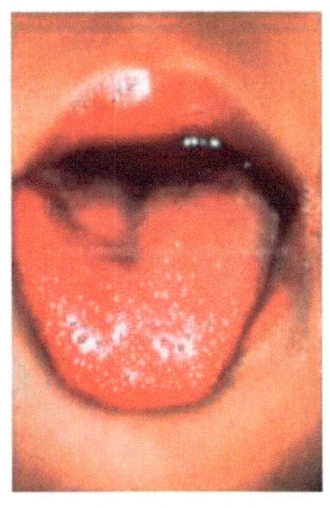 "Strawberry tongue"	Scarlet fever, Kawasaki disease, toxic shock syndrome
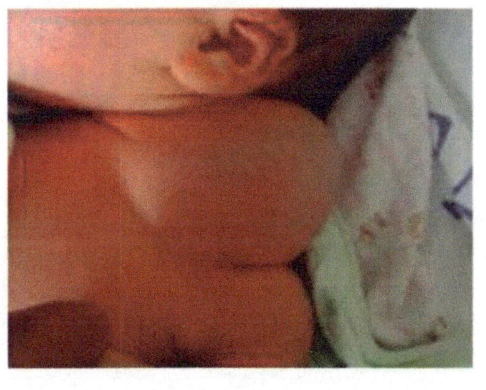 Streak ovaries, congenital heart disease, horseshoe kidney, cystic hygroma at birth*, short stature, webbed neck, lymphedema	Turner syndrome (45,XO)

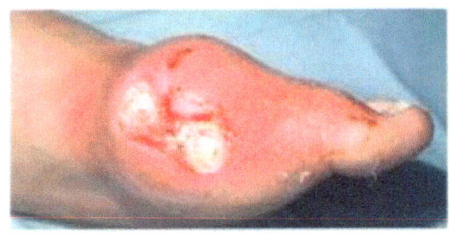

Gout/podagra (hyperuricemia)

Sudden swollen/painful big toe joint, tophi

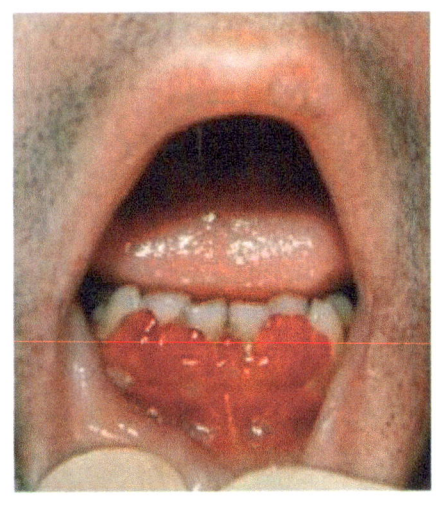

Scurvy (vitamin C deficiency: can't hydroxylate proline/lysine for collagen synthesis)

Swollen gums, mucosal bleeding, poor wound healing, petechiae

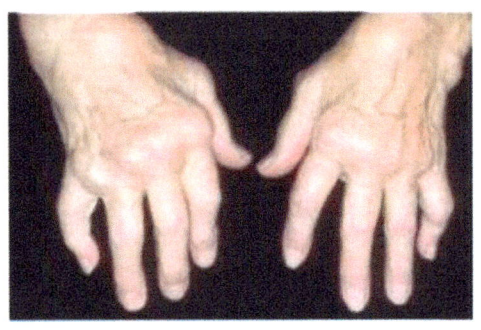

Osteoarthritis (osteophytes on PIP [Bouchard nodes], DIP [Heberden nodes])

Swollen, hard, painful finger joints

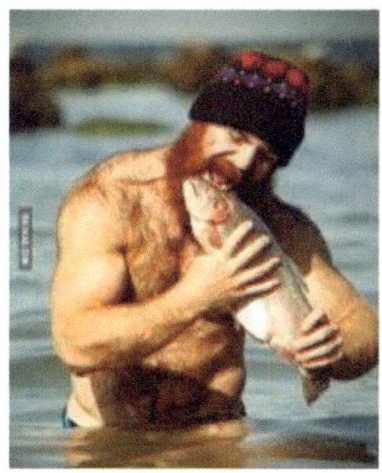

Thyroid and parathyroid tumors, pheochromocytoma

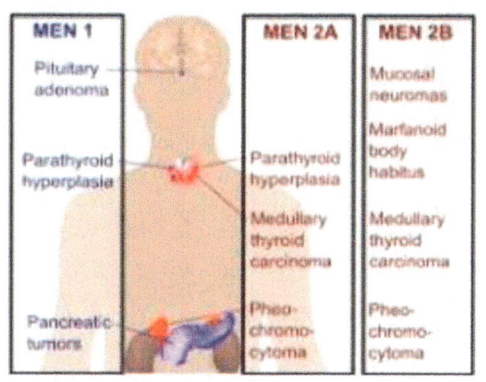

MEN 2A (autosomal dominant ret mutation)

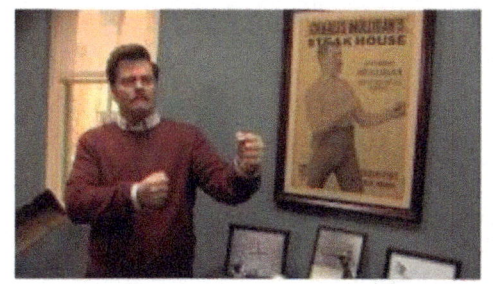

Thyroid tumors, pheochromocytoma, ganglioneuromatosis

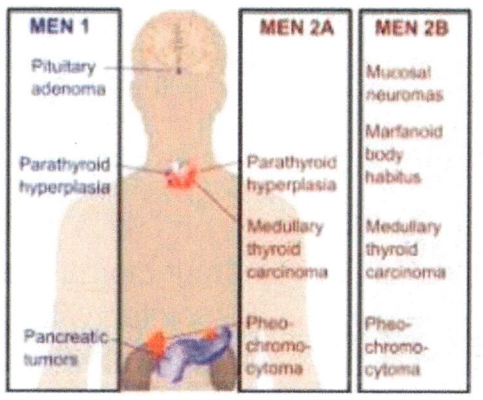

MEN 2B (autosomal dominant ret mutation)

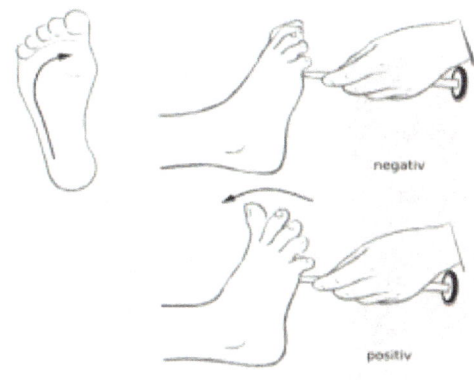

Toe extension/fanning upon plantar scrape

Babinski sign (UMN lesion)

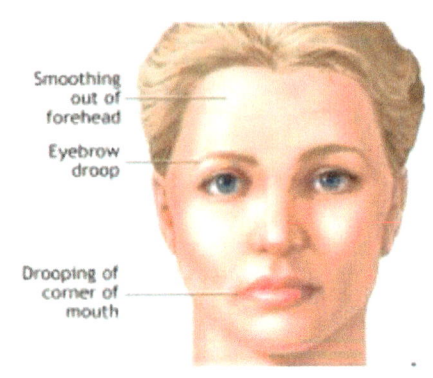 Unilateral facial drooping involving forehead	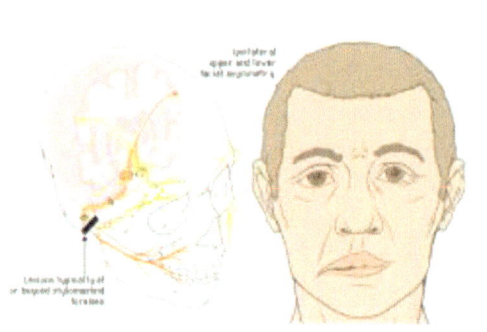 Facial nerve (LMN CN VII palsy)
Urethritis, conjunctivitis, arthritis in a male	Reactive arthritis associated with HLA-B27
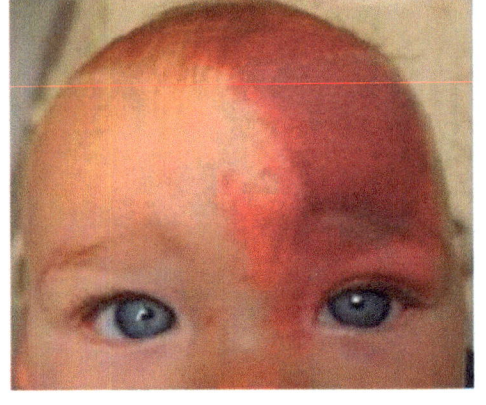 Vascular birthmark (port-wine stain)	Hemangioma (benign, but associated with Sturge-Weber syndrome)
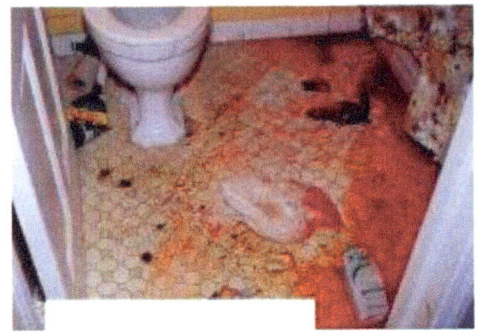 Vomiting blood following gastroesophageal lacerations	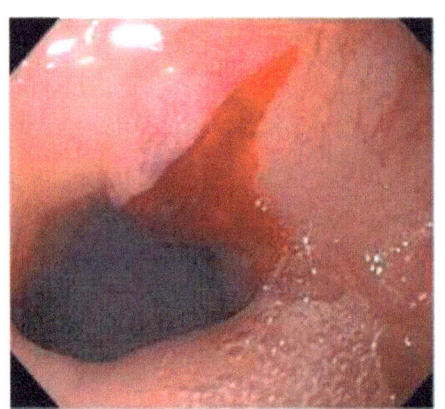

	Mallory-Weiss syndrome (alcoholic and bulimic patients)
Weight loss, diarrhea, arthritis, fever, adenopathy	Whipple disease (Tropheryma whipplei)
"Worst headache of my life"	Subarachnoid hemorrhage

Section 4

High-Yield Review

Mastering High Yield Topics for USMLE Step 1: Elite Strategies

Given its extensive syllabus and the crucial role it plays in a medical student's career, preparing for the USMLE Step 1 can be intimidating. Fortunately, you can increase the effectiveness and efficiency of your preparation by concentrating on High Yield Topics for USMLE Step 1 and comprehending the 80/20 rule. According to this theory, roughly 80% of the material you would encounter on the test can be represented by 20% of the study materials. You may optimize your study time and raise your score by concentrating on these high-yield subjects.

Understanding how content is distributed across different medical topics and disciplines is essential. According to the official USMLE website, the exam content specifications, physician tasks and competences, and discipline specifications are broken down in depth in the tables below. These percentages are intended to help students successfully focus their study efforts and show the variety of content that may be anticipated in each category. Remember that these percentages could vary, which emphasizes how crucial it is to frequently check the official website for updates in order to be aware of any changes.

Step 1 Test Content Specifications- High Yield Topics for USMLE Step 1

System**	Range, %
Human Development***	1-3
Blood & Lymphoreticular/Immune Systems	8–13
Behavioral Health & Nervous Systems/Special Senses	10–14
Musculoskeletal, Skin & Subcutaneous Tissue	7–12
Cardiovascular System	6-11
Respiratory & Renal/Urinary Systems	10–15
Gastrointestinal System	5–10
Reproductive & Endocrine Systems	9–13
Multisystem Processes & Disorders	11-16
Biostatistics & Epidemiology/Population Health	4–6
Social Sciences: Communication and Interpersonal Skills	6–9

From the official USMLE website, usmle.org

* The percentages could change at any time. * The distribution of foundational science material among the organ systems is determined by the diagnosis and course of the condition.

*** Normal Age-Related Findings and Care of the Well Patient are included in the Human Development subject. Depending on the diagnosis or course of the condition, the remaining content from the General Principles category has been divided among the various organ system categories.

Step 1: High Yield Topics for the USMLE Physician Tasks/Competencies Specifications*

Competency	Range, %*
Medical Knowledge: Applying Foundational Science Concepts	60–70
Patient Care: Diagnosis	20–25
History/Physical Examination	
Diagnosis	
Communication and Interpersonal Skills	6–9
Practice–based Learning & Improvement	4–6

The percentages could change at any time.

Step 1: High Yield Subjects for the USMLE Discipline Specifications*

Discipline	Range, %
Pathology	44–52
Physiology	25–35
Pharmacology	15–22
Biochemistry & Nutrition	14–24
Microbiology	10–15
Immunology	6–11
Gross Anatomy & Embryology	11–15
Histology & Cell Biology	8–13
Behavioral Sciences	8–13
Genetics	5–9

* The percentages could change at any time.

Following the summary of the USMLE Step 1 content requirements, it's equally critical to focus on particular high-yield subjects that are essential for the best possible exam preparation. The important topics in each medical specialty that are usually given higher weight on the test are listed in this section.

Anatomy

1. Cranial Nerves and Cerebral Lobes: Emphasis on recognizing images and comprehending signs of malfunction.
2. Nerves and Dermatomes: Crucial for the diagnosis of disorders associated with spinal cord injury.
3. Understand the lymph nodes' discharge patterns, particularly with regard to malignancies.
4. Discover the typical brachial plexus lesions and how they manifest.
5. Radiology of the Thorax and Abdomen: Know how to recognize organs and diseases on CT images.
6. Recognize the vascular supply and prevalent dysfunctions in the genitourinary and pelvic floor systems.
7. In tests, watershed areas are essential for identifying ischemia damage.

Physiology

1. action potentials, Recognize the phases particularly in cardiac and brain cells.
2. Lung and Heart Volumes: Learn to decipher graphical data.
3. Understand the changes in the hemoglobin dissociation curve and their clinical implications.
4. GI Hormones: Pay attention to how hormone abnormalities affect the gastrointestinal tract.
5. Renal Physiology: An in-depth examination of common diseases and nephron function.
6. Sarcomeres: Research the mechanics of muscle contraction; frequently examined using electron microscope images.

Biochemistry

1. Metabolic Pathways: Stress knowledge of enzymatic flaws and how they affect the body as a whole.
2. Vitamin Deficiencies: Commonly evaluated are important vitamins such as A, B1, B3, B9, B12, C, and D.
3. Genetic Disorders: Pay particular attention to conditions such as lysosomal storage diseases, glycogen storage diseases, and galactosemia.

Microbes and Contagious Illnesses

1. Classification of Bacteria and Viral Agents: Recognize the morphological and genetic characteristics that are essential for identifying diseases.
2. Fungi & Parasites: Focus on high-yield pathogens like giardia and malaria.
3. Know the typical symptoms and treatments of infection syndromes, particularly in children and patients with weakened immune systems.

Pharmacology

1. Drug Mechanisms and Side Effects: Crucial for chemotherapy, antivirals, and antibiotics.
2. Understand the main medications and their significant side effects, including antiretrovirals and antipsychotics.

Pathology

1. Understand the fundamental pathological mechanisms behind numerous disease states, including cell injury and death.
2. Questions about autoimmune disorders and the healing process are frequently directly related to inflammation and repair.

Integration Based on Systems

1. Cardiovascular and Pulmonary Diseases: Common ailments include COPD, asthma, and myocardial infarction.
2. Neurological Disorders: Pay particular attention to neurodegenerative illnesses, multiple sclerosis, and stroke.
3. Gastrointestinal Conditions: High-yield diseases include hepatic disorders and inflammatory bowel disease.
4. Endocrine and Metabolic Disorders: Adrenal diseases, thyroid issues, and diabetes are important.

Biostatistics and Social Sciences

1. Healthcare Delivery: Recognize the many kinds of insurance and preventative care.
2. Biostatistics: The ability to analyze study data, comprehend biases, and comprehend study design.

A fundamental component of the USMLE Step 1 exam is each of these domains. You may maximize your study time and improve your exam performance by concentrating on these high-yield subjects. Keep in mind that practice problems are crucial for comprehending how these subjects are assessed and for applying theoretical knowledge to real-world situations. I wish you luck as you get ready!

Basic Principles and Tips

Although we all hope that we will never need first aid, accidents can happen. Knowing how to react can make all the difference in situations ranging from minor accidents like cuts and burns to more serious emergencies. We'll go over the fundamentals of first aid in this article and provide some quick fixes for typical situations.

Fundamentals of First Aid

You might just have a few seconds to respond in an emergency. Understanding the acronym DRABC is essential for rapid thinking. You can use this information to help you navigate those crucial first stages. What does DRABC signify, then?

- **D for Danger:** Make sure you and the injured person are in a safe area before approaching them. This can entail, for instance, turning off electrical equipment or relocating the person away from traffic.
- **R for Response:** To determine whether the injured person is responding and thinking clearly, speak to them calmly and plainly. If they don't seem cognizant, give them a little shake or tap to see if they react.
- **A for Airway:** If the victim is not responding, check their airway. To make sure there is no obstruction, tilt their head back and open their mouth.
- **B for Breathing:** Pay attention to your breathing and feel it. Start CPR if their breathing is irregular.

- **C for Circulation:** Look for life-giving symptoms like coughing or movement. Proceed with CPR if none is discovered.

As soon as you've completed the DRABC checks, make an emergency assistance call.

Advice for Typical First Aid Situations

Abrasions and Cuts

Among the most frequent injuries are minor cuts and scrapes. Usually, these may be handled at home.

- Use flowing water and mild soap to gently clean the wound.
- If the cut is bleeding, apply little pressure with gauze or a clean cloth.
- Use an antiseptic lotion, like Neosporin, as soon as the bleeding has stopped.
- Apply bandages and give the wound careful attention.
- Should the wound continue to drain or bleed, clean it frequently and replace the bandage.

Keep an eye out for symptoms of infection, such as fever, edema, extreme redness, or discharge. Get medical help immediately if you think an infection is possible.

Scalds and Burns

In most cases, first-degree burns can be treated at home.

- Apply cool running water to the burn for 10 to 15 minutes to relieve it right away. (Applying ice straight to the skin can exacerbate the damage.)
- Aloe vera or burn cream can be applied to the burn to soothe the skin. Verify that the product is intended for treating burns.
- Cover the burn with a sterile gauze bandage. Securely but loosely wrap it.
- To aid with any pain, take over-the-counter medications like ibuprofen.
- Look for any indications of infection on the burn.

Get medical help right away if your burn is more severe, such as a second or third degree burn.

Choking

A typical household risk, particularly for kids, is choking. As choking is always an emergency, it needs to be treated right away to prevent unconsciousness or worse.

- Check the airway first. Check to see if they can cough or talk.
- Use the Heimlich technique if the person's airway is closed. It could take multiple tries before you are able to open the airway.
- Dial 911 right away if you are unable to clear the airway or if the person stops responding.

A person who is choking should not have their back smacked since this may force the obstruction farther down their airway.

Bleeding noses

In most cases, nosebleeds are fairly small injuries that don't require medical attention.

- Ask the person to pinch their nose while sitting up straight. (Verify that their breathing is still possible.)
- To prevent them from swallowing blood, which could cause vomiting, have them lean forward a little.
- Check to see if the bleeding has stopped after five minutes. Otherwise, repeat this procedure for five more minutes.
- While pinching the nose shut, think of placing a cold pack to it.

Seek medical help if the nosebleed persists and causes significant blood loss. This is particularly crucial if the person starts to feel faint or lightheaded.

Strains and Sprains

Use the RICE approach (rest, ice, compression, and elevation) for sprains and strains.

- Give the wounded area some rest.
- To lessen swelling, apply ice.
- Apply a bandage that is compressed.
- To reduce inflammation, raise the affected limb.

Bites of Animals

Animal bites, particularly those from dogs or wild animals, can quickly cause infection. Immediate action is necessary to prevent this.

- Use soap and water to clean the wound.
- Use an antibacterial lotion.
- To apply pressure and stop the bleeding, use a fresh cloth or gauze pad.
- Seek medical attention right once, especially if the animal is unknown or wild, as rabies immunization may be required.

Passing out

Rarely is fainting by itself harmful. However, if a person strikes their head or sustains other injuries in a fall, it could result in serious injury.

- Encourage someone to sit down and put their head below their knees if they are experiencing lightheadedness or vertigo.
- Make sure they are lying down and raise their legs if they have already passed out.
- After they come to, maintain them in a supine position for a few minutes before gradually assisting them in sitting up.
- Provide them with a meal or beverage.
- Keep an eye out for any issues with breathing, speaking, or thinking clearly.

Seek medical assessment to rule out any serious underlying illnesses if the reason of fainting is not immediately obvious, such as dehydration.

The poisoning

There are many potentially harmful items in the typical home. Depending on the drug in question, poisoning symptoms can vary greatly. Treating the issue yourself is usually not a good idea if someone has consumed, breathed, or come into touch with a dangerous material. Instead, get advice right away by contacting Poison Control or emergency services.

Eye Damage

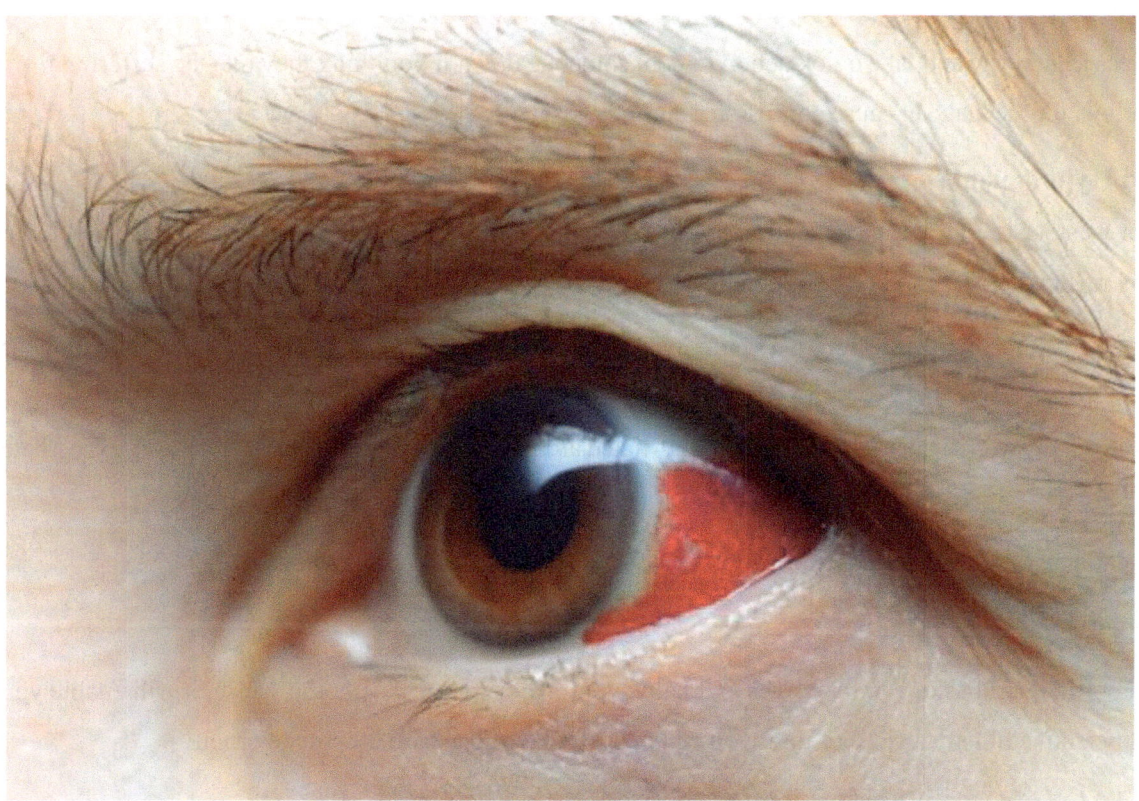

Injuries to the eyes can be particularly unpleasant and frightening.

- Encourage the person to blink or use an eye wash station to rinse their eyes with water if they are exposed to little irritants like dust or sand.
- Do not try to remove a foreign object or chemical that has become lodged in the eye. Get medical help right away and cover the eye with a fresh cloth or cup without applying pressure.

Dislocations and Fractures

Unfortunately, fractured or dislocated bones are a somewhat common injury.

- You should not attempt to realign the bone yourself if you suspect a fracture or dislocation.
- Use garments or blankets to support the damaged region and keep it as still as possible.
- To reduce swelling, wrap cloth-wrapped cold packs around the wound.
- As soon as you can, get medical help.

Heat Stroke and Heat Exhaustion

Particularly for those who work outside, heat-related illnesses pose a serious risk during hot or muggy weather. Action must always be taken right away in this scenario.

- Take someone to a cooler location, like a building or a shaded area, if you see them exhibiting signs of heat exhaustion.
- Offer them water.
- If at all possible, cover their body with cold, moist towels.
- Keep an eye on them to gauge their level of recovery.

Call emergency services right away and take quick action to cool someone down if you think they may be suffering from heat stroke, a more serious illness that can cause confusion, fainting, or seizures.

Both Frostbite and Hypothermia

Just as harmful as hot weather is cold weather. Both frostbite and hypothermia are dangerous illnesses that need to be treated immediately by raising the victim's body temperature.

- To treat hypothermia, transfer the person to a warm location, cover them with blankets, or warm them with your body heat.
- To treat frostbite, apply warm water—not hot—to the afflicted area. Avoid rubbing the area as this may exacerbate the damage.

Do not try to finish treatment on your own in any situation. Get medical help as soon as you can.

Be Ready for Anything

A basic understanding of first aid basics can save lives and help avoid major injuries. If nothing else, it will enable you to care for a wounded person until help arrives or until you can take them to the closest emergency room.

We hope that this advice has given you a better understanding of how to handle an injury. For additional information and better direction, we advise taking a certified first-aid training course if you'd like to learn more.

If someone else's carelessness causes harm to you or a loved one, you should be fairly compensated. You can acquire it with our aid.

Mnemonics and Memory Aids

Clinical practice necessitates a solid understanding of a vast and intricate body of knowledge. When attempting to remember information that needs to be memorized, such the results of a physical examination or the causes of specific diseases, mnemonics and other memory aids can be useful. The following list of mnemonics can be useful.

Common Systolic Heart Murmurs to Remember:

- Aortic
- Stenosis
- Systolic

- Mitral
- Regurgitation
- Physiologic (also called functional systolic flow murmur, a heart murmur heard without cardiac abnormalities)

During systole, all of the aforementioned murmurs can be heard.

The Most Valuable Player honor goes to MR PASS.

- Prolapse,
- valve,
- mitral

As an additional systolic murmur, add MVP.

MS ARD and MR PASS frequently hang out together.

- The diastolic,
- aortic,
- mitral,
- stenosis phases
- Diastole

all of the aforementioned murmurs are audible.

Symptoms of Aortic Stenosis

A person may have SAD if they have clinically severe aortic stenosis.

- Syncope
- Angina
- Dyspnea

Physiologic S2 Heart Sound Split

The aortic and pulmonic components of the second heart sound can be heard independently, which is a typical observation. Most toddlers and adults exhibit this finding, but it becomes less prevalent after the age of 55. The degree of split increases with inspiration and decreases with expiration, and is produced by a delay in the pulmonic component.

Tactile or vocal fremitus: increases as tissue density (i.e., the region of lung consolidation in pneumonia) increases.

For the Etiology of Delirium: DELIRIUMS

- Drugs: Any time a new medicine is prescribed or the dosage is changed. Anticholinergics (tricyclic antidepressants, first-generation antihistamines), neuroleptics (halo peridol, among others), opioids (especially meperidine), long-acting benzodiazepines (diazepam, clonazepam), alcohol, and other drugs are particularly problematic.
- Emotional (depression, loss), electrolyte imbalance

- Low PO2 (hypoxemia from pulmonary embolus, MI, chronic obstructive pulmonary disease, pneumonia), and abstinence from drugs (giving up alcohol and other addictive substances)
- Infection: The most frequent cause of delirium is either pneumonia or a urinary tract infection.
- Decreased sensory input (darkness, deafness, changes in environment), retention of pee or feces
- Ictal or postictal state: One of the most frequent causes of a single seizure in an older adult is alcohol withdrawal.
- Undernutrition includes dehydration, particularly surgical volume disruption, vitamin B12 or folate insufficiency, and protein/calorie malnutrition.
- Metabolic (ill-managed diabetic mellitus, hypo- or hyperthyroidism that is ignored or undertreated), and cardiac (myocardial infarction, heart failure, dysrhythmia) issues
- Subdural hematoma: Owing to atrophy and fragile vasculature, this condition may arise from relatively small head trauma to the brain.

Urinary incontinence causes that can be treated include: DIAPERS

- Delirium
- Urinary infection
- Drugs (diuretics, etc.)
- psychological conditions (depression)
- atrophic urethritis and vaginitis
- High urine production (heart failure, hyperglycemia from undiagnosed or inadequately managed diabetes mellitus)
- Limited freedom of movement
- Impaction of the stool

Anticholinergic Overdose or Misuse Presentation

Tricyclic antidepressants (amitriptyline [Elavil], nortriptyline [Pamelor]) and first-generation antihistamines (diphenhydramine [Benadryl], chlorpheniramine [Chlor-Trimeton], etc.) are examples of drugs with strong anticholinergic effects.

When a patient abuses or overdoses on drugs that have strong anticholinergic effects, they may be:

- Dry as a bone (dry mouth)
- Blind as a bat (blurred vision)
- Flushing red as a beet
- Bewildered as a hatter
- The condition known as hyperthermia
- Inability to see (visual abnormalities);
- inability to urinate (retention of urine);
- inability to perform actions that rhyme with "spittle," constipation

It should be noted that an older patient who has taken a first-generation antihistamine, an over-the-counter sleep aid that contains diphenhydramine (Benadryl),

any medicine known to have strong anticholinergic effects may exhibit a milder version of these findings.

Acute pancreatitis causes include: I'm smashed.

- Idiopathic (believed to be caused by microlithiasis or a hypertensive sphincter)
- Gallstones, which often pass through the common bile duct and lodge in the Vater's ampulla.
- Ethanol (typically excessive alcohol consumption)
- Injury (often a blunt abdominal injury)
- Systemic corticosteroid usage, or steroids
- Paramyxovirus, which causes mumps, as well as Epstein-Barr and cytomegalovirus
- Autoimmune conditions (systemic lupus erythematosus, polyarteritis nodosa)
- Certain snake bites and scorpion stings
- ERCP (after endoscopic retrograde cholangiopancreatography)
- Hyperlipidemia, including hypertriglyceridemia and hyponatremia;
- Hypercalcemia
- Medication (NSAIDs, azathioprine, sulfonamides, didanosine, DDP-4 inhibitor [-gliptin], diuretics [loop and thiazide], and duodenal ulcers

Healthcare Mnemonics: A Cautionary Note

I must offer a warning even if these memory aides are beneficial. Treatment mnemonics can be troublesome since the learner may have learned the steps to do by heart, but they may not fully understand the benefits of a certain intervention. Understanding the "why" in addition to the "how" is essential for safe therapeutic practice.

USMLE Step 1 Sample Questions And Answers

First Aid for Diseases, Disorders, Deficiencies, and Syndromes (USMLE Step 1)
Q. Adenosine deaminase (ADA) Deficiency

One kind of SCIDs and an immunodeficiency condition are brought on by an inherited mistake in adenine metabolism. Both B and T cells are destroyed by the buildup of adenine.

A rise in dATP has lymphotoxic effects.

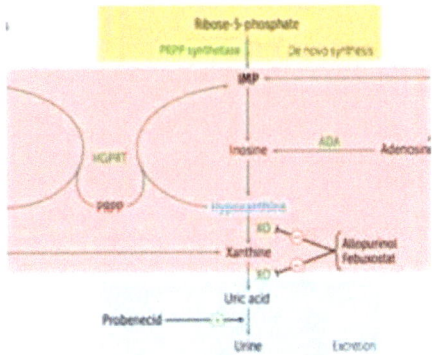

Q. The Lesch-Nyhan condition

Absence of HGPRT, which changes guanine into GMP and hypoxanthine into IMP, results in defective purine salvage. causes de novo purine synthesis and excessive uric acid production.

Recessive X-linked

Results: gout, dystonia, hyperuricemia (orange "sand" [sodium urate crystals] in diaper), violence, self-mutilation, and intellectual impairment.

Treatment options include febuxostat or allopurinol (2nd line).

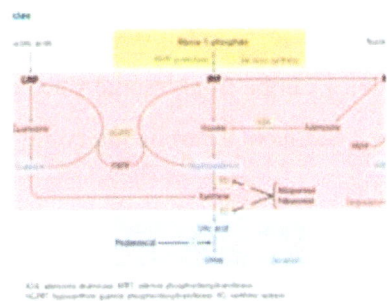

Q. The Bloom Syndrome

caused by BLM gene mutations that result in the production of a mutant DNA helicase protein

Short stature, a propensity for cancer development, and genetic instability are characteristics of a rare autosomal recessive condition.

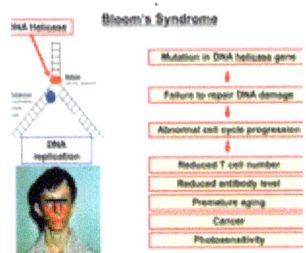

Q. Xeroderma Pigmentosum (XP)

Defect of Nucleotide Excision Repair

Due to exposure to UV light, the defect hinders the repair of pyrimidine dimers.

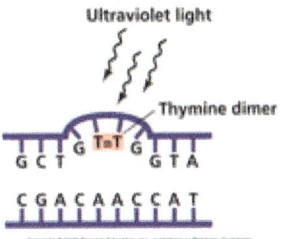

Q. (Hereditary Nonpolyposis Colorectal Cancer) Lynch Syndrome

Defective mismatch correction

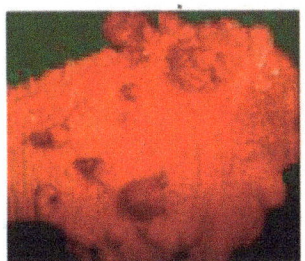

Q. Ataxia Telangiectasia

Defect of nonhomologous end joining

Cell cycle arrest is caused by defects in the ATM gene, which prevent DNA double strands from being repaired.

IgA deficiency, spider angiomas (telangiectasia), and cerebellar abnormalities (ataxia) make up the triad.

elevated AFP.

reduced levels of IgA, IgG, and IgE.

neurological atrophy and lymphopenia.

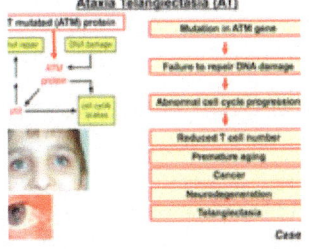

Q. Fanconi anemia

Defect of nonhomologous end joining

Q. I-cell disease (also known as mucolipidosis type II or inclusion cell disease)

Lysosomal storage disease that is inherited

Proteins are secreted extracellularly instead of being transported to lysosomes when the Golgi fails to phosphorylate mannose residues (i.e., mannose-6-phosphate) on glycoproteins due to a defect in N-acetylglucosaminyl-1-phosphotransferase.

causes elevated plasma levels of lysosomal enzymes, clouded corneas, limited joint movement, and coarse facial characteristics.

Children are frequently deadly.

Q. Zellweger syndrome

Mutations in the PEX genes cause an autosomal recessive disease of peroxisome biogenesis.

causes hepatomegaly, hypotonia, convulsions, and premature death.

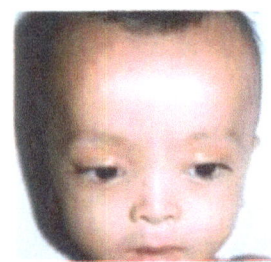

Q. **Disease of Refsum**

Alpha oxidation (peroxisome) autosomal recessive disorder: phytanic acid not converted to pristanic acid

causes the fourth toe to shorten, ataxia, cataracts or night blindness, scaly skin, and epiphyseal dysplasia.

Tx: plasmaphoresis, diet

Q. Adrenoleukodystrophy (ALD)

High levels of saturated very-long-chain fatty acids (VLCFAs) are connected to demyelination of the neurological system and malfunction of the adrenal cortex, an X-linked disorder of beta oxidation (peroxisome).

causes an accumulation of VLCFAs in the brain's white matter, testes, and adrenal glands.

Chronic illness that can cause death, coma, and adrenal gland crisis

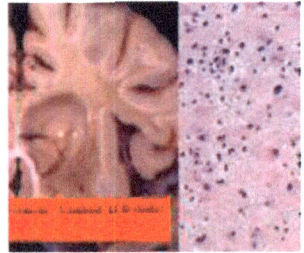

Q. (The primary ciliary dyskinesia) Kartagener syndrome

A deficiency in the dynein arm causes immotile cilia.

increases the likelihood of an ectopic pregnancy and causes infertility in both males and females as a result of immotile sperm and malfunctioning fallopian tube cilia, respectively.

recurrent sinusitis, situs inversus, and bronchiectasis (for example, dextrocardia on CXR = Defect in left-right Dynein can lead to Dextrocardia).

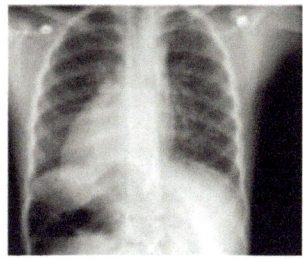

Q. Imperfect Osteogenesis

Brittle bone disease, a genetic bone ailment, is brought on by a number of gene abnormalities, most frequently COL1A1 and COL1A2.

The most prevalent variety is autosomal dominant and produces type I collagen in a normally normal manner. Type III is the worst; it is perinatally fatal.

The following are possible symptoms: -Several fractures with little damage that could happen during childbirth

-The translucent connective tissue covering the choroidal veins causes blue sclerae.

-Abnormal ossicles, or hearing loss

-Teeth abnormalities in certain forms include opalescent teeth that wear down quickly because of a lack of dentin (dentinogenesis imperfecta).

Tx: Bisphosphonates are used to reduce the risk of fractures.

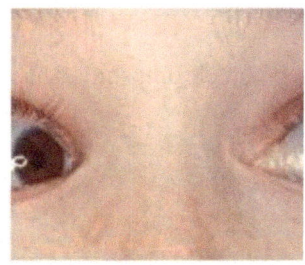

Q. Ehlers-Danlos Syndrome (EDS)

Hypermobile joints, a propensity to bleed (easy bruising), and hyperextensible skin are all symptoms of defective collagen synthesis.

several kinds. Severity and inheritance differ.

either recessive or autosomal dominant.

may be linked to organ rupture, berry and aortic aneurysms, and joint dislocation.

The most prevalent kind is hypermobility (joint instability).

Type V collagen (COL5A1, COL5A2) mutations produce the classical type (joint and skin symptoms) and I

Lack of type III collagen in the vascular type (vascular and organ rupture)

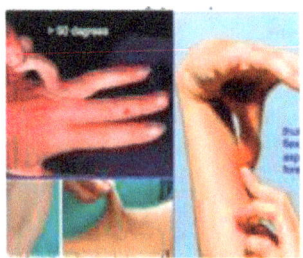

Hypermobility Type: Ehlers-Danlos Syndrome

most prevalent kind of EDS.

Q. Ehlers-Danlos syndrome: Classical form of symptoms related to the joints and skin

EDS brought on by a mutation in type I and type V collagen (COL5A1, COL5A2)

Q. **The syndrome of Ehlers-Danlos: Vascular kind (both organ rupture and vascular)**

Type III collagen deficiency causes EDS.

Q. Menkes disease

X-linked recessive connective tissue disorder brought on by a malfunctioning Menkes protein (ATP7A), which impairs copper transport and absorption. reduces lysyl oxidase activity (copper is a required cofactor).

causes hypotonia, growth retardation, and brittle, "kinky" hair.

Q. The Marfan syndrome

Autosomal dominant CT disease that affects the heart, eyes, and skeleton

Defective fibrillin, a glycoprotein that surrounds elastin, is caused by a mutation in the FBN1 gene on chromosome 15.

Findings:

- tall with lengthy limbs
- excavum or pectus carinatum
- hypermobile joints
- arachnodactyly, or long, tapering fingers and ties
- aortic cystic medial necrosis
- aortic incapacity
- identifying aortic aneurysms
- floppy mitral valve
- lens subluxation (temporal and upward)

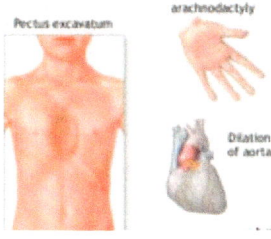

Q. The McCune-Albright syndrome

Traditional Mosaicism

An activating mutation in the G-protein/CAMP/adenylate cyclase signaling pathway causes the condition.

characterized by early puberty, endocrine problems, Cafe-au-lait patches, and fibrous dysplasia of the bone.

Mutations that impact all cells before fertilization are fatal, however mosaicism patients can survive.

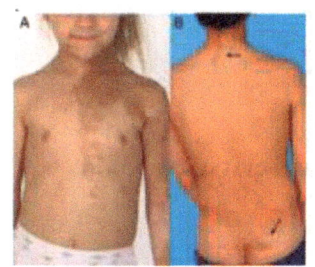

Q. Prader-Willi Syndrome

Imprinting (Maternal hushed, paternal deleted)

Maternal imprinting occurs when the paternal gene is altered or deleted and the maternal gene is typically quiet.

connected to a deletion or mutation of paternal chromosome 15

causes hypogonadism, hypotonia, obesity, hyperphagia, and intellectual impairment.

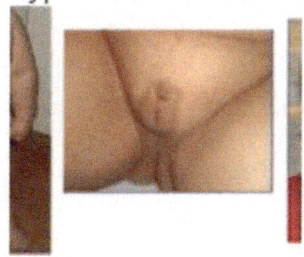

Q. Angelman Syndrome

Imprinting (paternal silent, maternal deleted)

Paternal imprinting occurs when the mother's gene is altered or deleted and the father's gene is typically silent.

connected to chromosome 15's maternal copy's UBE3A gene mutation or deletion

causes severe intellectual impairment, ataxia, seizures, and inappropriate laughter ("happy puppet").

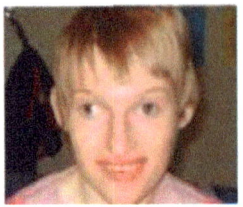

Q. Vitamin D-resistant rickets (hypophosphatemic)

Rickets, are inherited and X-linked. Phosphate wasting at the proximal tubule is caused by the dominant disease.

results in a presentation akin to rickets

Q. Leigh Syndrome, also known as subacute necrotizing encephalopathy

is a progressive neurodegenerative disease that typically manifests in early childhood and has a characteristic neuropathology that leads to death within two years.

-MtDNA mutations -Respiratory complex I or IV mutations that occur often.

The mitochondrial-encoded pyruvate dehydrogenase complex is mutated in the X-linked variant.

-Affects the central nervous system; breathing irregularities, dystonia, movement problems, and cystic cavitation.

-The survivors have mental retardation.

Q. Mitochondrial Myopathies (MELAS)

Mutations in mtDNA

Rare conditions frequently manifest as CNS illness, lactic acidosis, and myopathy.

secondary to oxidative phosphorylation's failure. Red fibers are ragged in the biopsies.

One such instance is MELAS, which includes lactic acidosis, stroke-like events, and mitochondrial encephalopathy.

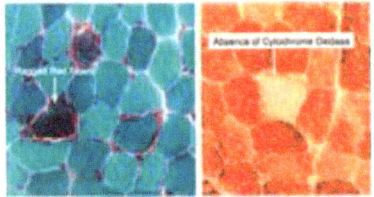

Q. Leber's Hereditary Optic Neuropathy (LHON)

Mitochondrial DNA disorder

caused by point mutations in the cytochrome reductase gene, which permits electrons to move from cytochromes b and c1 to cytochrome c.

Patients with subacute bilateral loss of central vision are mostly men in their 20s and 30s. Typically, permanent

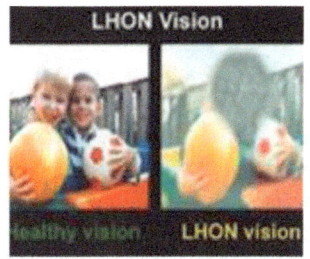

Q. Cystic Fibrosis

Recessive Autosomal

protein structural defect in the CFTR gene on chromosome 7; typically, Phe508 is deleted. The most prevalent fatal genetic illness in the Caucasian population

An ATP-gated Cl− channel that is encoded by CFTR secretes Cl− in the GI tract and lungs and reabsorbs it in sweat glands. The most frequent mutation results in a misfolded protein, which keeps the protein in the RER instead of moving it to the cell membrane, reducing the secretion of Cl− (and H2O). Increased intracellular Cl− causes an increase in H2O reabsorption, which in turn causes an unusually thick mucus to be released into the GI tract and lungs.

Sweat containing (> 60 mEq/L) is diagnostic. ECF H2O/Na+ losses and associated renal K+/H+ squandering can produce contraction alkalosis and hypokalemia.

Rise in immunoreactive trypsinogen (screening for newborns)

Chronic bronchitis and bronchiectasis, recurrent lung infections (e.g., S aureus [early infancy], P aeruginosa [adolescence]), Meconium ileus in neonates, biliary cirrhosis, liver illness, fat-soluble vitamin deficiencies, pancreatic insufficiency, and malabsorption with steatorrhea Subfertility in women (amenorrhea, excessively thick cervical mucus) and infertility in men (lack of vas deferens, spermatogenesis may be unaffected). Nasal polyps and nail clubbing

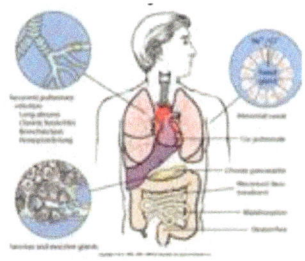

Q. Achondroplasia

Dominant Autosomal

Inhibition of chondrocyte proliferation occurs when fibroblast growth factor receptor 3 (FGFR3) is mutated.

Leg length has a greater impact on dwarfism than head or torso size.

Complete penetration

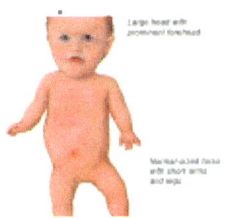

Q. Autosomal Dominant of the Polycystic Kidney Disease

Dominant Autosomal

Multiple big cysts cause the kidneys to expand massively on both sides.

PKD1 (chromosome 16) mutations account for 85% of cases, with PKD2 (chromosome 4) mutations accounting for the remaining instances.

most prevalent inherited reason for adult renal failure. The diagnosis is aided by a favorable family history and a large number of kidney and liver cysts, which are often discovered by the third or fourth decade of life.

Q. (FAP) familial adenomatous polyposis

Dominant Autosomal

After puberty, adenomatous polyps blanket the colon. Unless the colon is removed, it develops into colon cancer.

Chromosome 5q (APC gene) mutations; five letters in "polyp."

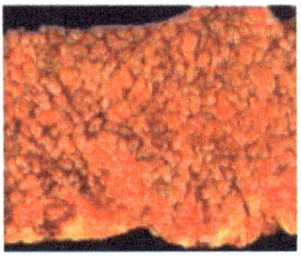

Q. Hypercholesterolemia Family

Dominant Autosomal

elevated LDL because of a malfunctioning or nonexistent LDL receptor.

causes tendon xanthomas (usually in the Achilles tendon), corneal arcus, and significant atherosclerosis disease early in life.

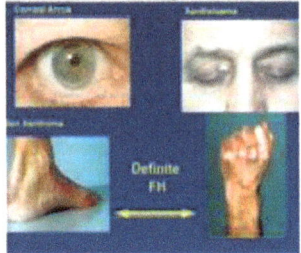

Q. Herited Hemorrhagic telangiectasia (Osler-Weber-Rendu syndrome)

Dominant Autosomal

blood vascular disease that is inherited.

Results: recurring epistaxis, skin discolorations, arteriovenous malformations (AVMs), hematuria, GI bleeding, and branching skin lesions (telangiectasias).

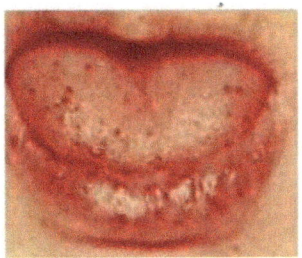

Hereditary Spherocytosis

Autosomal Dominant

Hemolytic anemia; spectrin or ankyrin-defective sphenodrocytes

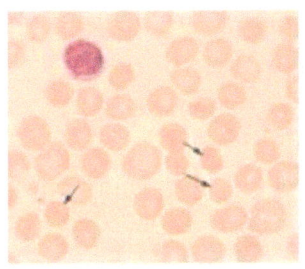

Q. (CAG) Huntington's disease

Dominant Autosomal

The trinucleotide repeat disorder gene on chromosome 4 is CAG.

Results: caudate atrophy, choreiform movements, sadness, and gradual dementia.

reduced GABA, decreased ACh, and increased dopamine in the brain.

shows anticipation: a rise in recurrences corresponds to a fall in the age of initiation.

Q. Li-Fraumeni Syndrome

Dominant Autosomal

TP53 abnormalities result in several early-stage cancers.

The SBLA cancer syndrome (sarcoma, breast, leukemia, and adrenal gland) is another name for it.

Q. (MEN) Multiple Endocrine Neoplasia.

Dominant Autosomal

hereditary tumors of endocrine glands, including as the pituitary, thyroid, adrenal medulla, parathyroid, and pancreas, are a feature of several different syndromes (1, 2A, and 2B).

The MEN1 gene is linked to MEN 1.

RET gene is linked to MEN 2A and 2B.

Q. Type 1 neurofibroma (von Recklinghausen illness)

Variable expression, 100% penetrance, autosomal dominant.

Café-au-lait spots and cutaneous neurofibromas are hallmarks of this neurocutaneous condition.

caused by changes in chromosome 17's NF1 gene; the 17 letters in "von Recklinghausen."

Q. Type 2 neurofibromatosis

dominated by autosomal

Results: ependymomas, meningiomas, bilateral acoustic schwannomas, and juvenile cataracts

On chromosome 22, the NF2 gene

Q. Tuberculosis Sclerosis

dominated by autosomal

A neurocutaneous condition that affects multiple organ systems and is typified by a large number of benign hamartomas. Expression that is variable

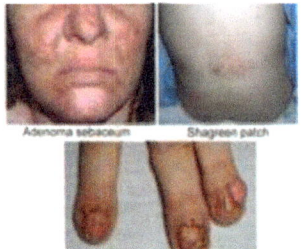

Q. von Hippel-Lindau Disease

dominated by autosomal

illness marked by the growth of many tumors, both benign and malignant

connected to the loss of the tumor suppressor gene VHL on chromosome 3 (3p).

For chromosome 3, von Hippel-Lindau is equivalent to three terms.

Q. Duchenne Muscular dystrophy

Deleted dystrophin, X-linked recessive

Muscle regeneration is impeded due to shortened dystrophin protein caused by frameshift or nonsense mutations.

The pelvic girdle muscles are the first to become weak, and this weakness spreads superiorly.

Calf muscular pseudohypertrophy brought on by fibrofatty muscle replacement.

Gower maneuver: patients stand up with the assistance of their upper extremities. waddling motion. begins before the age of five. One prevalent cause of mortality is dilated cardiomyopathy.

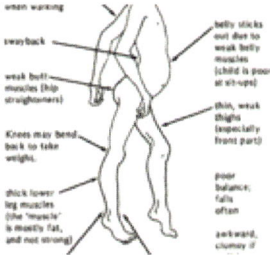

Q. Becker muscular dystrophy

Non-frameshift X-linked recessive

Nonframeshift insertions in the dystrophin gene (partially functioning rather than truncated) are usually the cause of X-linked disorders.

beginning in early adulthood or adolescence

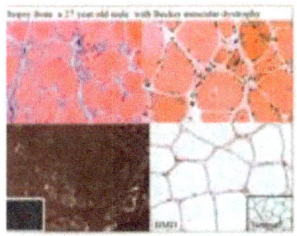

Q. Myotonic Muscular Dystrophy Type 1 (CTG)

dominated by autosoma

Expansion of the CTG trinucleotide repeat in the DMPK gene = aberrant myotonin protein kinase expression = myotonia, frontal baldness, cataracts, muscular atrophy, and arrhythmia

"My Tonia, My Testicles (testicular atrophy), My Toupee (frontal balding), My Ticker (arrhythmia)"

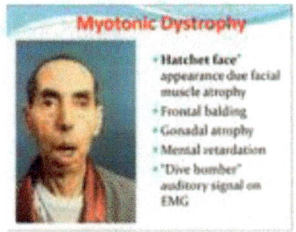

Q. The Rett Syndrome

Normal early development is followed by a loss of intentional hand usage, characteristic hand movements, slower brain and head growth, atypical gait, seizures, and mental retardation. This neurodevelopmental sporadic disorder typically affects children aged 1-4.

De novo mutations of MECP2 on the X chromosome are the cause of the majority of cases.

Almost primarily affects women; it is a component of autism spectrum disorders.

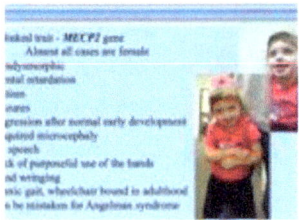

Q. (CGG) fragile X syndrome

Dominant inheritance associated to X

*FMR1 gene trinucleotide repeat = methylation = expression decline.

After Down syndrome, it is the second most prevalent cause of hereditary intellectual disability.

Findings include autism, mitral valve prolapse, a long face with a wide jaw, large everted ears, and postpubertal macroorchidism (enlarged testes).

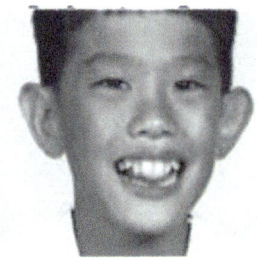

Q. Friedrich Ataxia (GAA)

-Early Childhood

-degenerative disease of the cerebellum and several tract lesions of the spinal cord

-appearance of ATAXIA (cerebellum) with loss of proprioception and vibratory sensation, LE muscle weakness, and DTR

The FRATAXIN gene's unstable trinucleotide repeat (GAA) is autosomal recessive and crucial for the regulation of mitochondrial iron; if it is disrupted, free radical damage occurs through the fentin reaction.

-occurs during early childhood

Hypertrophic cardiomyopathy (a/w)

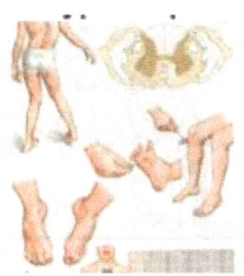

Q. Down Syndrome (Trisomy 21)

Flat faces, pronounced epicanthal folds, a single palmar wrinkle, a gap between the first two toes, duodenal atresia, Hirschsprung disease, congenital heart disease (ASD), and Brushfield spots are all signs of intellectual disability. C-21, which codes for the amyloid precursor protein, is linked to early-onset Alzheimer's disease and raises the risk of AML and ALL.

Meiotic nondisjunction accounts for 95% of instances. Unbalanced Robertsonian translocation, usually between chromosomes 14 and 21, accounts for 4% of instances.

The most prevalent cause of hereditary intellectual disability and the most prevalent viable chromosomal condition

Ultrasound in the first trimester typically reveals:

- ➢ -Increase nasal bone hypoplasia and nuchal translucency
- ➢ Reduce blood levels of PAPP-A
- ➢ -Raise free β-hCG levels.

The quad screen of the second trimester displays

- ➢ Reduction of α-fetoprotein
- ➢ -A rise in β-hCG
- ➢ -A reduction in estriol
- ➢ A rise in the hormone inhibin A

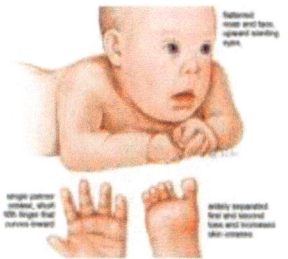

Q. Edwards Syndrome (trisomy 18)

Congenital heart disease, low-set ears, clenched hands with overlapping fingers, rocker-bottom feet, micrognathia (small jaw), and a prominent occiput are all signs of severe intellectual handicap. Usually, death happens within a year of birth.

The second most frequent trisomy that results in a live birth

Initial trimester:

- A reduction in PAPP-A
- Reduction in free β-hCG

Quad-screen:

- A reduction in α-fetoprotein
- Decreased normal inhibin A, estriol, or β-hCG.

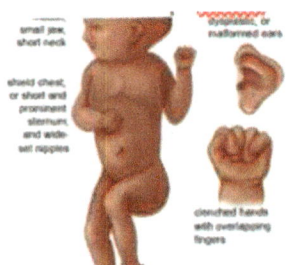

Q. Patau Syndrome (trisomy 13)

Microphthalmia, microcephaly, cleft lip/palate, holoProsencephaly, polydactyly, congenital heart disease, severe intellectual handicap, rockerbottom feet, and cutis aplasia. Usually, death happens within a year of birth.

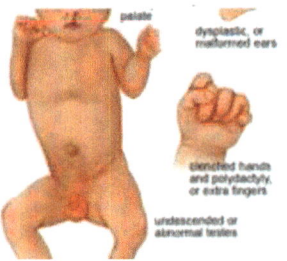

Q. Syndrome of Cri du Chat

Congenital short arm chromosome 5 microdeletion (46,XX or XY, 5p-)

Microcephaly, epicanthal folds, high-pitched wailing or meowing, moderate to severe intellectual impairment, and heart abnormalities (VSD) were among the findings.

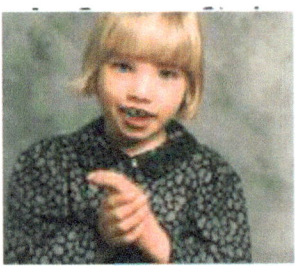

Q. The Williams Syndrome

Congenital microdeletion of chromosome 7's long arm, which includes the elastin gene.

Results include a unique "elfin" appearance, intellectual impairment, hypercalcemia (heightened sensitivity to vitamin D), highly developed verbal abilities, a high degree of sociability toward strangers, and cardiovascular issues (renal artery stenosis, supravalvular aortic stenosis).

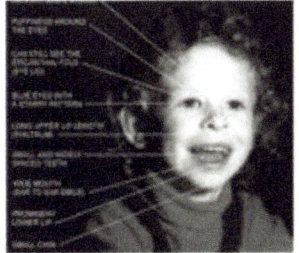

Q. 22q11 deletion Syndromes

CATCH-22

Heart problems, thymic aplasia, cleft palate, aberrant facial features, and hypocalcemia brought on by parathyroid aplasia

22nd chromosome

DiGeorge syndrome: cardiac, parathyroid, and thymic abnormalities

Defects of the palate, face, and heart are known as velocardiofacial syndrome.

Q. The DiGeorge Syndrome

absence of the thymus and T-cell insufficiency due to the third and fourth pharyngeal pouches not developing

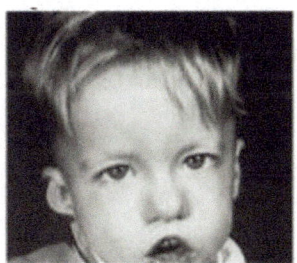

Q. Velocardiofacial Syndrome

Autosomal genetic disease

Chromosome 22 part (22q11.2)

- Soft palate cleft, humorous face
- A baby has trouble feeding (milk comes out of the nose).

- Elongated face, almond eyes, tiny ears, and wide nose
- Aortic conditions
- Delayed mental development

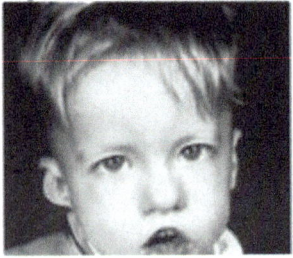

Q. Scurvy

Gum bleeding, weakness, loose teeth, and damaged capillaries beneath the skin are symptoms of a vitamin C deficient condition.

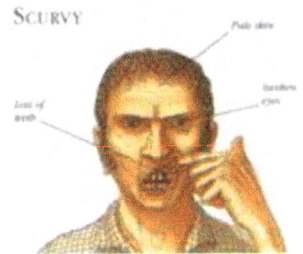

Q. Wernicke-Korsakoff Syndrome

Long-term heavy alcohol consumption can cause organic brain syndrome, which manifests as disorientation, incomprehensible speech, and impaired motor coordination.

It might be brought on by a lack of thiamine, a vitamin that heavy drinkers have trouble metabolizing.

* The classic triad (ataxia, confusion, and ophthalmoplegia) plus confabulation, personality abnormalities, and irreversible memory loss

harm to the mammillary bodies and the thalamic medial dorsal nucleus

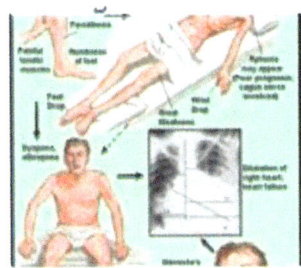

Q. Dry beriberi

Polyneuritis, symmetrical muscular atrophy, and thiamine deficiency

Q. Wet beriberi

Thiamine (deficiency in vitamin B1). polyneuropathy, edema, and dilated cardiomyopathy.

Q. Pellagra

illness caused by a lack of niacin. The "4 D's"—diarrhea, dermatitis, dementia, and death—are among the symptoms.

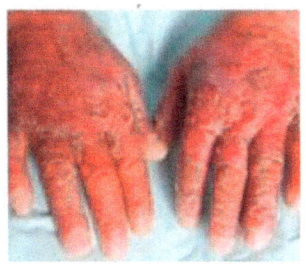

Q. The Hartnup disease

Neurtal aminoiaciduria, decreased absorption from the stomach, decreased tryptophan conversion to niacin, and pellagra are all symptoms of autosomal recessive disease, which is characterized by diminished neutral amino acid (such as tryptophan) transporters on PCTs and enterocytes.

Treat with niacin and a high-protein diet.

Q. Kwashiorkor

a pediatric chronic malnutrition condition where a lack of protein increases a child's susceptibility to various illnesses like influenza, diarrhea, and measles.

Malnutrition of proteins

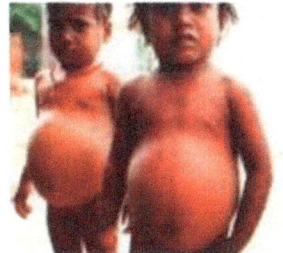

Q. Marasmus

Early infancy is a time of severe protein-calorie malnutrition, which causes growth to stop, bodily structures to deteriorate, and the newborn to eventually pass away.

Muscle atrophy

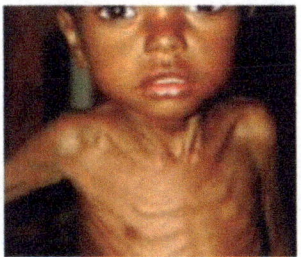

Q. Pyruvate Dehydrogenase Deficiency

causes pyruvate to accumulate, which is then converted to alanine (by ALT) and lactate (by LDH).

acquired or X-linked (Vit B deficiency, arsenic poisoning)

Lactic acidosis, neurologic abnormalities, and elevated serum alanine beginning in infancy

TX: Consume more ketogenic nutrients, such as more fat or more leucine and lysine.

Q. Glucose 6-Phosphate Dehydrogenase

This is the most prevalent enzyme deficiency in humans. more common in African Americans. Boost resistance to malaria.

Glutathione must be kept decreased by NADPH in order to detoxify peroxides and free radicals.

Hemolytic anemia results from a decrease in RBC NADPH because of inadequate RBC defense against oxidizing agents or pathogens.

Oxidative stress causes denatured hemoglobin, or Heinz bodies, to form inside red blood cells.

Bite cells are produced when splenic macrophages phagocytically remove Heinz bodies.

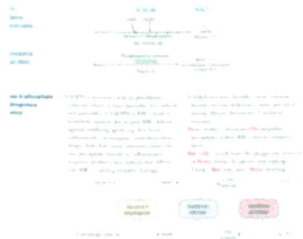

Q. Fructosuria essential

*Fructokinase defect

Recessive autosomal *

harmless and asymptomatic

*Fructose is not confined within cells.

Fructose is converted to fructose-6-phosphate* mostly by hexokinase.

Fructose can be found in urine and blood.

Fructose metabolism disorders that are less severe than galactose metabolism disorders

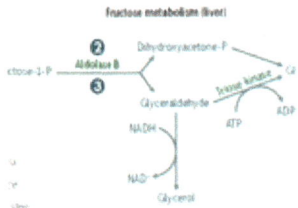

Q. Intolerance to Fructose

Aldolase B def. AR.

When F1P builds up, phosphate is produced, which leads to glycogenolysis and gluconeogenesis and hypoglycemia.

Consuming fruit, juice, or honey might result in cirrhosis, jaundice, vomiting, and hypoglycemia.

The urine dipstick, which solely checks for glucose, will come back negative.

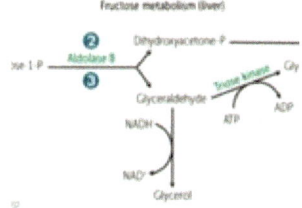

Q. Galactokinase deficiency

Galactokinase deficiency that is autosomal recessive.

If galactose is consumed, galactitol builds up.

When the baby starts eating, symptoms appear (lactose in breast milk and regular formula).

Symptoms include infantile cataracts and galactose in the blood (galactosemia) and urine (galactosuria). may manifest as an inability to follow objects or a lack of social smiles.

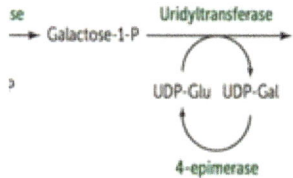

Q. Classic galactosemia

Patients who are homozygous for a faulty galactose-1-phosphate uridyltransferase gene have an autosomal recessive illness.

The buildup of harmful compounds, such as galactitol, which builds up in the eye's lens, causes damage.

Jaundice, hepatomegaly, infantile cataracts, intellectual impairment, and inability to thrive are some of the symptoms.

can cause neonatal E. Coli sepsis.

Therapy: cut off lactose and galactose (galactose plus glucose) from your diet.

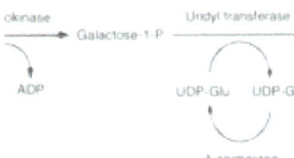

Galactose metabolism

Q. Lactase deficiency

absence of the brush border enzyme that breaks down lactose, a disaccharide, into its constituent monosaccharides (galactose and glucose).

First, people of Asian, African, or Native American heritage frequently experience age-dependent deterioration beyond childhood due to the lack of the lactase-persistent gene.

Secondary: brush boundary loss brought on by autoimmune diseases, gastroenteritis (such as rotavirus), etc. Rare congenital lactase deficiency caused by a faulty gene

With the lactose hydrogen breath test, the pH of the stool decreases and the hydrogen content of the breath increases.

flatulence, cramping, bloating, and osmotic diarrhea.

Q. Deficiency of N-acetylglutamate synthase

Carbamoyl synthetase I requires this cofactor; its absence results in hyperammonemia and elevated ornithine with normal urea cycle enzymes.

appears in newborns as inadequate eating, intellectual impairment, developmental delay, and poorly controlled breathing and body temperature.

Similar to how carbamoyl phosphate synthetase I deficiency manifests

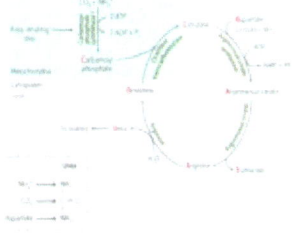

Q. Deficiency of ornithine transcarbamylase

The most prevalent urea cycle disorder is an X-linked recessive illness. It hinders the body's capacity to expel ammonia and is frequently noticeable in the first few days of life, though it can also appear later.

The pyrimidine synthesis route converts excess carbamoyl phosphate to orotic acid.

Results: elevated blood and urine orotic acid, hyperammonemia symptoms, and a drop in BUN

*Anemia without megaloblastic (as opposed to orotic aciduria)

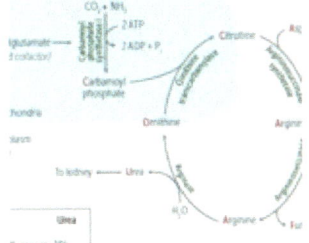

Q. (PKU) phenylketonuria

Large amounts of the amino acid phenylalanine build up due to an autosomal recessive disorder that causes growth retardation, seizures, intellectual incapacity, fair skin, dermatitis, and musty body odor (disorder of aromatic amino acid metabolism).

Because of the decline in the cofactors for tetrahydrobiopterin (malignant form) or phenylalanine hydroxylase

Phenylacetate, phenyllactate, and phenylpyruvate are phenylketones.

Aspartame, an artificial sweetener, must be avoided.

Q. (PKU) Maternal

Phenylketone buildup during pregnancy due to improper nutritional therapy

Microcephaly, intellectual impairment, growth retardation, and congenital cardiac abnormalities were discovered in the infant.

Q. (MSUD) maple syrup urine disease

Recessive autosomal

Reduced branched-chain α-ketoacid dehydrogenase (B1) results in blocked breakdown of branched amino acids (isoleucine, leucine, and valine), which raises blood levels of α-ketoacids, particularly leucine.

causes pigment-forming homogentisic acid to build up in tissue, which leads to severe CNS abnormalities, intellectual incapacity, mortality, vomiting, poor feeding, and urine that smells like maple syrup or burnt sugar.

- ➢ * Ochronosis (bluish-black sclerae and connective tissue)
- ➢ Prolonged exposure to air causes urine to turn black.
- ➢ Debilitating arthralgias (cartilage-toxic homogentisic acid).

Treatment consists of dietary restrictions for isoleucine, leucine, and valine as well as thiamine supplements.

Q. Ochronosis (alkaptonuria)

Congenital homogentisate oxidase impairment in the tyrosine-to-fumarate degradation pathway

Benign, autosomal recessive illness

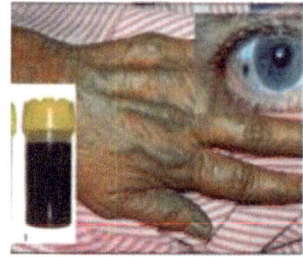

Q. **The homocystinuria**

Types:

- Deficiency in cystathione synthase
- decreased pyridoxal phosphate affinity of cystathione synthase
- Deficiency in methionine synthase (homcysteine methyltransferase)

Homocysteine elevation in the urine, osteoporosis, inward and downward lens subluxation as opposed to marfan, thrombosis, marfanoid, and intellectual disability

Tx: pyridoxine

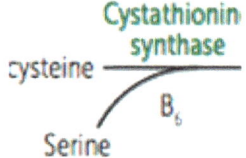

Q. **Cystinuria**

Defective transport of cystine, ornithine, arginine, and lysine across the intestinal and renal tubular epithelium is the cause of this AR recessive illness.

When there is too much cystine in the urine, it precipitates out and forms hexagonal cystine crystals, which causes recurrent nephrolithiasis.

The test for urine cyanide-nitroprusside is diagnostic. Treatment: chelating drugs like penicillamine and urine alkalinization (such potassium citrate and acetazolamide) make cystine stones more soluble; stay well hydrated.

Q. **Von Gierke decrease (GSD type I)**

The enzyme glucose 6 phosphatase is deficient.

Glycogen: regular structure and high glycogen concentration in the liver and kidney

- Severe hypoglycemia while fasting
- A rise in liver and kidney glycogen results in hepatonephromegaly.
- Raise blood lactate (acidemia) levels
- Raise TGs
- A rise in uric acid

Always treat with raw corn or starch; avoid fasting metabolism.

Q. (Type II GSD) Pompe disease

Alpha-1,6-glucosidase activity of lysosomal acid maltase (1-4 glucosidase) is a deficient enzyme.

Glycogen: normal cytosolic content, lysosomal buildup in the heart, muscle, and liver

Most severe in infants, cardiomegaly, myopathy, hepatomegaly, hypotonia, neuromuscular disease, and NO hypoglycemia

destroys the PumP (muscle, liver, and heart).

Q. (Type III GSD) Cori disease

Also known as limit dextrinosis and Forbes disease

Alpha-1,6-glucosidase debranching enzyme deficiency: 4:4 transferase activity

Glycogen: excessive and aberrant cytosolic levels of limit dextrin-like structures

Muscular dystrophy can result from hepatomegaly, cardiomyopathy, muscle weakness, hypotonia, and MILD hypoglycemia.

Q. McArdle Disease (type V GSD)

Deficiency in skeletal muscle glycogen phosphorylase (Myophosphorylase)

An increase in muscle glycogen that the muscle is unable to digest is unpleasant.

cramping in the muscles, myoglobinuria (red urine) following intense exercise, and arrhythmia due to electrolyte imbalances. Muscular blood flow during exercise causes the second-wind effect.

No rise in lactate levels, but an increase in CK. Usually, blood glucose levels remain unchanged.

Q. Fabry Disease

Sphingolipidoses (XR is the only one)

The enzyme α-galactosidase A is deficient.

Substrate accumulated: Ceramide trihexoside

Findings:

-Early: Hypohidrosis, angiokeratomas A, and episodic peripheral neuropathy.

-Late: cardiovascular disease, progressive renal failure.

Q. Tay-Sachs Disease

AR, or sphingolipidoses

Hexosaminidase A is an enzyme that is lacking.

Substance accumulated: GM2 ganglioside

Results:

-Delays in development due to progressive neurodegeneration

The macula's "cherry-red" spot

-Onion-skin lysosomes

There is no hepatosplenomegaly.

Q. Metachromatic Leukodystrophy

AR, or sphingolipidoses

Enzyme Deficit: Arylsulfatase A

Cerebroside sulfate is the accumulated substrate.

Findings:

-Death and ataxia due to central and peripheral demyelination

Q. (Globoid cell leukodystrophy) Krabbe disease

AR, or sphingolipidoses

The enzyme galactocerebrosidase is deficient.

Accumulated substrate: psychosine galactocerebroside

Results: Globoid cells, peripheral neuropathy, developmental delay, and optic atrophy

Q. (Glucocerebrosidase deficiency) Gaucher disease

AR, or sphingolipidoses

Glucocerebrosidase (β-glucosidase) is a deficient enzyme.

Substrate accumulated: glucocerebroside

Findings:

Most typical

However, hepatosplenomegaly

-Pancytopenia

Osteoporosis

-Femur aseptic necrosis

-Crisses of the bones

-__?__ cells (macrophages loaded with lipids that resemble crumpled tissue paper)

Q. Niemann-Pick illness

AR, or sphingolipidoses

Sphingomyelinase is an enzyme that is lacking.

Substance accumulated: Sphingomyelin

Findings:

-Degeneration of the neurons

-Hepatosplenomegaly

-Foam cells (macrophages loaded with lipids)

The macula's "cherry-red" spot

Q. (MPS I) Hurler Syndrome

AR, or mucopolysaccharides

The enzyme α-l-iduronidase is deficient.

Heparan sulfate and dermatan sulfate are examples of accumulated substrate.

Findings:

-A delay in development

-Gargoylism

-Obstruction of the airway

-Clouding of the cornea

-Hepatosplenomegaly

Q. (MPS II) Hunter Syndrome

XR, or mucopolysaccharides

Iduronate sulfatase is an enzyme that is lacking.

Heparan sulfate and dermatan sulfate are examples of accumulated substrate.

Findings:

-A delay in development

-Gargoylism

-Obstruction of the airway

-NO clouding of the cornea

-Hepatosplenomegaly

-Aggressive conduct

Q. **Systemic primary carnitine deficiency**

Toxic buildup in the cytosol due to an inherited malfunction in the transport of LCFAs into the mitochondria causes hypoglycemia, hypotonia, and weakness

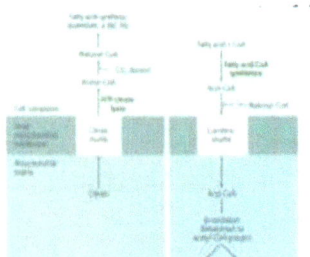

Deficiency of medium-chain acyl-CoA dehydrogenase

Reduced capacity to convert fatty acids into acyl-CoA due to an AR dysfunction of fatty acid oxidation results in the buildup of 8- to 10-carbon fatty acyl carnitines in the blood and hypoketotic hypoglycemia.

may manifest as coma, vomiting, lethargy, seizures, and liver dysfunction (Reye-like) in infancy or early childhood. prolonged physical therapy, elevated dicarboxylic acids in the urine, and subsequent carnitine insufficiency.

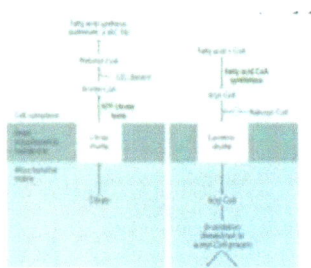

Q. **Deficiency of long-chain acyl CoA dehydrogenase**

Fatty acid oxidation disorder with reduced capacity to convert fatty acids into acyl-CoA --> hazardous buildup

Findings:

-Onset: infants

-Rhabdomyolysis and weakening of the muscles

-Arrhythmias and cardiomyopathy

-Hypoketotic low blood sugar

-Increased dicarboxylic acids in the urine

-The symptoms go away after medium chain TG treatment.

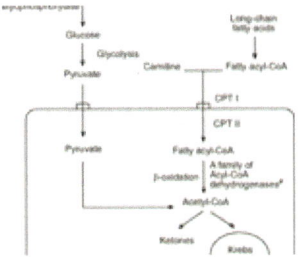

Q. Abetalipoproteinemia

Apolipoprotein B-48 and B-100 (Microsomal Transfer Protein; MTP gene) autosomal recessive deficiency

Infants with this condition exhibit significant fat malabsorption, steatorrhea, and underdevelopment.

Later symptoms include spinocerebellar degeneration brought on by vitamin A and *retinitis pigmentosa. RBC acathocytosis, progressive ataxia, and E deficiency

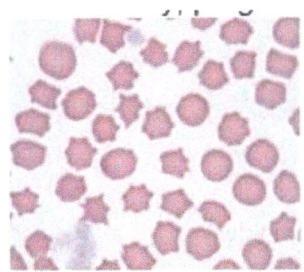

Q. (Type I) hyperchylomicronemia

AR

Apolipoprotein C-II or LPL deficiency

elevated TGs, cholesterol, and blood chylomicrons

Hepatosplenomegaly, eruptive/pruritic xanthomas, and pancreatitis (no risk for atherosclerosis). layer of creaminess in the supernatant

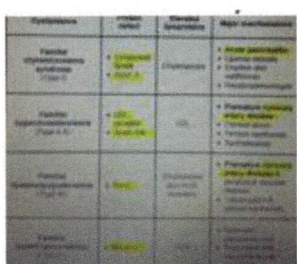

Q. (Type II) Familial Hypercholesterolemia

AD

Absence or deficiency of Apo B-100 or LDL receptors

↑ LDL, IIa cholesterol

↑ VLDL (IIb), cholesterol, and LDL

A heterozygote's cholesterol is approximately 300 mg/dL.

Very uncommon homozygotes have cholesterol levels of 700 mg/dL or more.

Achilles tendon xanthomas, ocular arcus, and accelerated atherosclerosis (may cause MI before age 20)

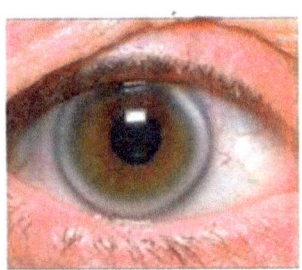

Q. (Type III) dysbetalipoproteinemia

AR

Apo E is flawed.

elevated chylomicrons and VLDL

Tuberoeruptive xanthomas, early atherosclerosis, and Striae palmaris (cholesterol in palmar wrinkles)

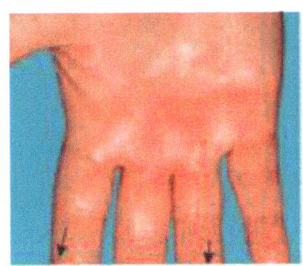

Q. (Type IV) hypertriglyceridemia

AD

VLDL overproduction in the liver

Higher VLDL and TGs (>1000)

Pancreatitis acute

Q. Type 1 of autoimmune polyendocrine syndrome

Whitaker syndrome, also known as APECED

An immune reaction directed against several endocrine organs, such as the pancreatic islets, adrenal glands, and parathyroids

Pathogenesis:

1. Thymic endothelial cells' inability to deliver endocrine antigens is caused by mutations in AIRE, which results in defective negative selection in the thymus.

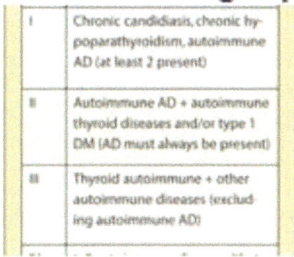

Q. IPEX syndrome (Immune dysregulation, X-linked, enteropathy, and polyendocrinopathy)

Uncommon x-linked illness

FOXP3 mutation equals lack of Tregs

enteropathy, polyendocrinopathy, and immunological dysregulation.

Q. Deficiency in early complement (C1-C4)

Deficiency in complement proteins:

increases vulnerability to type III hypersensitivity reactions and the risk of severe, recurring pyogenic sinus and respiratory tract infections. An elevated risk of SLE

Q. Deficiencies in terminal complement (C5-C9)

Deficiency in complement proteins:

makes one more vulnerable to recurring Neisseria bacteremia

Q. C1 esterase inhibitor deficiency

Because of the uncontrolled activation of kallikrein, it causes hereditary angioedema.

-ACE inhibitors should not be used.

characterized by declining C4 levels

Q. Paroxysmal nocturnal hemoglobinuria

A PIGA gene mutation that stops complement inhibitor anchors like DAF/CD55 and membrane inhibitor of reactive lysis (MIRL/CD59) from forming

RBC lysis mediated by complement

Q. (Bruton) X-linked agammaglobulinemia

-No B-cell maturation results from a mutation in the tyrosine kinase gene BTK.

-Recessive X-linked (in boys)

-After six months, recurrent enteroviral and bacterial infections (maternal IgG).

-Decreased Ig across all classes and absent B cells in peripheral blood.

-The tonsils and lymph nodes are absent or sparse.

Q. Selective IgA deficiency

The most prevalent immunodeficiency is 1°.

Most people are asymptomatic. able to identify autoimmune diseases, atopy, airway and gastrointestinal infections, and anaphylaxis to items containing IgA

Reduced IgA, Normal G, and M levels

Q. (CVID) common variable immunodeficiency

B-cell differentiation defect.

It may be significantly delayed and typically appears after the age of two. Risk factors include autoimmune disease, bronchiectasis, lymphoma, and sinopulmonary infections; can be acquired in the 20s and 30s.

Low immunoglobulins and plasma cells

Q. Thymic aplasia (DiGeorge syndrome)

deletion of -22q11; absence of the thymus and parathyroids; inability to build the third and fourth pharyngeal pouches.

-Recurrent viral/fungal infections (T-cell deficiency), tetany (hypocalcemia), and conotruncal abnormalities (e.g., truncus arteriosus, tetralogy of Fallot).

-Decrease Ca^{2+}, PTH, and T cells.

-CXR has no thymic shadow.

FISH found a loss at -22q11.

Q. IL-12 receptor deficiency

- reduced Th1 reaction. recessive inheritance.

-Disseminated fungal and mycobacterial infections, which could appear after receiving the BCG vaccine.

IFN-γ was reduced.

Q. Autosomal dominant hyper IgE syndrome (Job)

A STAT3 mutation-induced Th17 cell deficiency results in decreased neutrophil migration to infection sites.

FATED: retained primary teeth, IgE, cold (non-inflammatory) staphylococcal abscesses, coarse facial tissue, and dermatological issues (eczema).

IFN-γ reduced and IgE increased.

Q. Chronic Mucocutaneous Candidiasis (CMC)

collection of conditions when skin, nails, or mucous membranes become infected with the Candida fungus on a regular or persistent basis.

T-cell proliferation in vitro in response to Candida antigens is absent. lack of skin response to Candida antigens.

Q. (SCID) severe combined immunodeficiency

-A number of varieties, such as adenosine deaminase deficiency (autosomal recessive) and faulty IL-2R gamma chain (most prevalent, X-linked).

-Thrush, persistent diarrhea, and failure to thrive. recurring infections caused by bacteria, fungi, viruses, and protozoa.

-Bone marrow transplant (no rejection risk) is the treatment.

T-cell receptor excision circles (TRECs) have decreased.

-The absence of T cells (flow cytometry), germinal centers (lymph node biopsy), and thymic shadow (CXR).

Q. Hyper IgM syndrome is

X-linked recessive and most frequently caused by a CD40L deficiency on Th0 cells class switching defect.

Early-life severe pyogenic infections; opportunistic infections with CMV, Cryptosporidium, and Pneumocystis.

-Decreased IgG, IgA, and IgE by twofold, and increased IgM

Q. Wiskott-Aldrich syndrome

The X-linked recessive mutation in the WAS gene; T cells are unable to rearrange the actin cytoskeleton.

-Begins with recurring infections, eczema, and thrombocytopenic purpura.

-Raise the risk of cancer and autoimmune diseases.

-Return to normal levels of IgG and IgM. elevated IgE and IgA.

-A lesser number of platelets.

Q. leukocyte adhesion deficiency

A phagocyte's LFA-1 integrin (CD18) defect results in decreased chemotaxis and motility.

Frequent bacterial infections of the skin and mucous membranes, lack of pus production, poor wound healing, and delayed umbilical cord separation (> 30 days).

Neutrophils have increased. Neutrophils are absent from infection sites.

Q. Chediak- Higashi syndrome

The lysosomal trafficking regulator gene (LYST) is defective. Phagosome-lysosome fusion due to microtubule malfunction

Reciprocal autosomal

Infiltrative lymphohistiocytosis, peripheral neuropathy, progressive neurodegeneration, partial albinism, and recurrent pyogenic infections caused by streptococci and staphylococci.

giant granules in platelets and granulocytes. pancytopenia. mild flaws in coagulation.

Q. Chronic Granulomatous Disease (CGD)

A malfunction in NADPH oxidase and increases vulnerability to infections with organisms that produce catalase (Nocardia, Pseudomonas, Listeria, Aspergillus, Candida, E. Coli, Staphylococci, Serratia, B cepacia, and H pylori).

Most prevalent is X-linked recessive.

Dihydrorhodamine test abnormality (reduction in green fluorescence) (flow cytometry).

The nitroblue dye reduction test for tetrazolium is no longer valid.

Q. Patent Foramen Ovale

The inability of the fetal opening to ever seal results in an atrial septal defect, which is an opening in the septum that normally divides the atria.

may result in paradoxical emboli, which are venous thromboemboli that enter the circulation of systemic arteries.

Q. (PDA) patent ductus arteriosus

After birth, the ductus arteriosus fails to close, creating an irregular gap between the aorta and the pulmonary artery.

Section 5

Test-Taking Strategies

How To Overcome USMLE Step 1 Exam Anxiety

As medical students, getting ready for the USMLE Step 1 exam is one of the most stressful experiences we have. It's more than simply an exam; it has the power to influence our entire medical careers. The overwhelming pressure to do well might cause stress and anxiety, which can impair our readiness. But it is possible to overcome this anxiety, and I have discovered a number of techniques that have helped me control my dread and maintain my composure. I'll talk about what worked for me in this guide and offer some tips that can give you more self-assurance before taking the USMLE Step 1. Let's talk about overcoming exam anxiety for the USMLE Step 1.

Recognizing Step 1 Anxiety on the USMLE

Understanding what anxiety is and its causes is crucial before we can control it. The USMLE Step 1 assesses your mental stamina and strength in addition to your knowledge. Fear of failing, pressure to perform, and uncertainty about the exam's complexity are common causes of anxiety. For me, my worry was increased by the possibility that I wouldn't fit into a reputable residency program. I started to feel overwhelmed since I knew that the outcome may have a big effect on my future.

This anxiety might show up in a variety of ways. You may have panic episodes, difficulty focusing, or restless nights. It was a pervasive sense of uncertainty and fear for me. Even though I had performed well on my prior tests, I began to doubt my skills. The first step to conquering anxiety is realizing that it's normal and identifying the cause.

Creating a Practical Study Schedule

I overloaded my schedule in the beginning, which was one of my worst errors. I believed that studying for longer periods of time would inevitably produce better outcomes, so I tried to pack everything in as fast as possible. However, it only made me more anxious. For stress management, a realistic and well-organized study schedule is essential.

I started by dividing the content into digestible chunks and making a daily plan that wasn't too ambitious. I broke the material up into smaller themes rather than aiming for impractical objectives like studying a whole subject in a single day. Studying became less intimidating and more doable as a result. In order to refuel, I also made sure to include breaks and days off.

By following this methodical schedule, I was able to monitor my development without feeling hurried. I was able to observe noticeable progress every day, which in turn helped to lower my worry. You can control your preparation with a realistic strategy, which is crucial for reducing worry.

Avoid perfectionism and cultivate self-compassion.

As medical students, we frequently have unrealistic expectations of ourselves. I used to believe that I would flunk every practice test if I didn't receive a score of 90% or above. My stress level simply rose as a result of this meticulous mindset. I have to realize that it's acceptable to not know everything at once and learn to be kinder to myself.

Being self-compassionate entails acknowledging that everyone finds the USMLE Step 1 to be a challenging test. Making mistakes when preparing is OK because it's a necessary component of the learning process. I began to prioritize progress above perfection. I considered what I could learn and how I could get better rather than berating myself for a poor grade.

The secret to lowering worry is allowing oneself to be imperfect. Nobody expects you to be an all-knowing robot, after all. Changing my focus from unachievable perfection to consistent progress made me feel more relaxed and less anxious about how I performed.

Creating Good Study Practices

Creating good study habits was a key component in my ability to control my USMLE Step 1 anxiety. I quickly concluded that studying for extended periods of time without breaks wasn't effective. My anxiety increased as a result of my inability to recall information. I therefore modified my study strategy.

I started employing active learning strategies, like regularly completing practice questions, instructing others, and testing myself. This avoided burnout and made learning more interesting. Hours of reading or underlining were examples of passive studying, which frequently left me feeling frustrated since I didn't feel like I was getting anywhere. I felt more confident since I could see how much I was becoming better every day thanks to active learning.

I also made sure to get enough sleep, eat well, and exercise frequently. It may seem simple, but when you're anxious about an exam, it's simple to forget about these things. I started eating well-balanced meals, taking little walks during my breaks, and making sure I slept for at least seven hours every night. My energy levels and concentration significantly improved as a result of these adjustments.

Effective Time Management

An essential skill for USMLE Step 1 preparation is time management. The idea that there wasn't enough time to cover everything was one of the biggest causes of my anxiousness. I would frequently worry that I was lagging behind or that I wouldn't have enough time to complete the syllabus before the test.

Clearly defining priorities was essential to conquering this worry. I concentrated on high-yield themes and ones that I found most difficult rather than attempting to cover every single detail. I didn't let too many study materials divert me from using reliable resources like First Aid, UWorld, and Pathoma.

I also took care to give each task a precise time restriction. Even if I hadn't completed everything, I wouldn't allow myself to go over the allotted two hours for biochemistry. This helped me feel accomplished when I completed the next assignment and kept me from becoming bogged down in one topic for too long.

How to Handle Exam Day Nerves

I was anxious before the test day despite having spent months studying. It's quite normal to experience anxiety as the test draws near, but there are strategies to control these emotions so they don't affect how well you perform.

I made it a point to unwind as much as I could on the day before the test. Although it was difficult at first, I realized that cramming at the last minute wouldn't help, so I didn't study. Rather, I concentrated on eating a healthy dinner, getting a good night's sleep, and engaging in peaceful activities like reading a book or listening to music.

I told myself on test day that I had done my best to prepare and that the nervousness would pass quickly. Every time I felt my nerves getting the better of me, I used deep breathing techniques. I took brief breaks to stretch and decompress during the test. Exam day anxiety can be considerably decreased and optimal performance can be achieved by taking care of your physical and mental health.

Asking Mentors and Peers for Help

Asking for help was one of the best things I did as I was preparing for the USMLE Step 1. When you're anxious about an exam, it can feel lonely, but you're not alone. I discovered that everyone has anxiety after speaking with friends who were going through the same thing. When we were feeling low, we would encourage one another, discuss our hardships, and even trade advice.

I also asked mentors who had already completed the process for advice. It was very comforting to hear about their experiences and see how they coped with stress. They reminded me that anxiety is common and does not indicate a lack of skill. Do not be afraid to talk to someone about feeling overwhelmed. Just putting your worries into words can sometimes have a significant impact.

Meditation and Mindfulness Practices

Including meditation and mindfulness in my daily routine also helped me feel less anxious. I was skeptical at first because I believed I didn't have time for meditation. But I came to see that even five to ten minutes a day of mindfulness can have a significant impact on your mood.

I began practicing brief guided meditations and breathing techniques, especially on days when I was feeling really anxious. By doing this, I was able to keep my mind from racing with concerns about the future and instead remain focused and in the moment. Additionally, mindfulness helped me recognize when my thoughts were out of control and helped me to regain my composure.

Hours of meditation are not necessary to reap the rewards. You can approach your studies with greater clarity and less anxiety if you just set aside a little period of time each day to center yourself.

Acknowledging errors without dwelling on them

My fear of making mistakes was one of the main causes of my anxiety. I would feel like I was failing every time I answered a practice question incorrectly, which would make me anxious. But I had to come to terms with the fact that making mistakes is a necessary component of learning.

Instead of becoming disheartened when I made a mistake, I began to see it as a chance to get better. I would go over the question again and make sure I knew why I answered incorrectly. My anxiety decreased as a result of this mental change since I stopped viewing errors as a reflection of my skills. Rather, they served as stepping stones to material mastery.

Overcoming exam anxiety requires learning from errors without obsessing over them. It's critical to keep in mind that nobody has an ideal preparation process, and it's acceptable to make mistakes along the road.

Keeping a Positive Attitude and Visualizing Success

Lastly, visualizing is one of the most effective strategies for conquering anxiety. I neglected to envision what may go right because I was so preoccupied with what might go wrong. I began to picture myself entering the exam room composed, self-assured, and ready. I imagined that I would be able to clearly answer questions and feel proud of my work after I finished the test.

I was able to change my perspective from one of dread to one of confidence by envisioning success. I was able to lessen the negative ideas that exacerbated my anxiousness by concentrating on the positive results. It's critical to remind yourself that you are capable and that you can succeed if you have the correct mindset and adequate preparation.

Step 1 Anxiety on the USMLE Can Be Overcome

Although the USMLE Step 1 exam is unquestionably one of the most difficult medical school experiences, you don't have to be afraid of it. Although anxiety is a natural aspect of the process, it can be effectively managed by using the appropriate techniques. There are numerous strategies to reduce the stress related to this test, including developing a practical study schedule, engaging in self-compassion exercises, learning from errors, and asking for help.

Keep in mind that you are not traveling alone and that experiencing anxiety is normal. It's crucial that you act to control your worry so that it doesn't prevent you from succeeding. You can confidently take the USMLE Step 1 and emerge stronger if you have the correct attitude and strategy.

USMLE Candidates' Guide to Time Management: Effective Strategies

Academic knowledge is not enough to start the process of mastering the USMLE tests. It requires excellent time management abilities to guarantee a well-rounded, productive study schedule. In order to help USMLE candidates maximize their study time and achieve the ideal balance between learning and relaxation, we go into useful ideas in this book.

Comprehending the USMLE Task

For medical license in the US, passing the multi-step United States Medical Licensing Examination (USMLE) is essential. It assesses both medical knowledge and the capacity to use that information to provide patient care. Time management is an essential skill for all candidates because of the scope and depth of the material presented.

Making an Effective Study Schedule

Making a customized study schedule is one of the first stages to becoming an expert at time management. Depending on your skills and shortcomings, this plan should allot time for each subject. Keep in mind that flexibility is essential; as you work through your study material, your schedule should change to accommodate your changing demands.

Advice for a Successful Study Schedule

- Divide the study material into digestible portions.
- Establish clear objectives for every study session.
- To prevent burnout, incorporate brief breaks on a regular basis.
- Examine your schedule frequently and make any necessary adjustments.

Increasing the Effectiveness of Studying

Making every study session matter is more important than packing in more hours. This entails employing study strategies that improve comprehension and retention, like practice questions, active learning approaches, and recurring self-evaluation.

Reading Passively Is Not as Effective as Active Learning

It has been demonstrated that active learning, which entails interacting with the content through conversation, application, and questioning, is more successful than passive reading. Memory retention and comprehension can be greatly improved by employing strategies like mnemonics, flashcards, and teaching concepts to others.

Making Use of Superior Resources

Selecting the appropriate study resources is essential. Reputable resources provide thorough, current content that is in line with the goals and structure of the USMLE. Making use of these tools guarantees that you're learning the most pertinent content while also saving time.

Finding a Balance Between Study and Health

Finding a balance between study time and personal well-being is an essential part of time management. Maintaining the mental and physical endurance required for intense USMLE preparation requires regular exercise, a balanced diet, and enough sleep.

Making Good Use of Study Partners and Groups

Study partners and groups can help you prepare for the USMLE. They offer a forum for dialogue, elucidation of uncertainties, and reciprocal encouragement. To sustain productivity, make sure your study group is concentrated and that each session has clear goals.

Managing Your Time on Exam Day

Time management techniques are not limited to preparation; they also apply on test day. Practice with timed quizzes and practice exams, and become familiar with the format of the exam. This will enable you to efficiently manage your time throughout the actual USMLE, guaranteeing that you can respond to every question in the allocated period.

Frequent Evaluation and Self-Evaluation

Reviewing the content and evaluating your comprehension on a regular basis is crucial. This helps pinpoint areas that require additional attention in addition to reinforcing what has been learned. Make use of practice tests and self-assessment resources to monitor your development and modify your study schedule as necessary.

Using Technology to Study More Effectively

When it comes to USMLE preparation, technology can be a great ally. Utilize time management, scheduling, and flashcard apps. You can improve your preparation by using platforms, which include interactive materials and practice problems that closely resemble the USMLE format.

Preventing Typical Time Management Errors

Avoid typical mistakes include procrastinating, focusing too much on one subject at the expense of other subjects, and underestimating the amount of time needed for particular topics. You can steer clear of these obstacles and continue preparing for the USMLE by being aware of them.

In conclusion

One of the most important skills for USMLE applicants is effective time management. You may increase your study efficiency and success rate by making a customized study plan, utilizing active learning strategies, striking a balance between study and leisure time, and making use of top-notch resources. Keep in mind that passing the USMLE is a marathon, not a sprint. Make a good plan, study effectively, and feel confident when taking your tests.

FAQs

How can I make a USMLE study schedule that works?

Understanding your strengths and shortcomings, breaking the study material up into digestible portions, establishing clear objectives, and having the flexibility to modify your plan as necessary are all necessary for developing an efficient study schedule.

Which study strategies work best for the USMLE?

Flashcards, mnemonics, teaching concepts to others, and practice questions are examples of active learning strategies that work quite well for USMLE preparation.

To what extent does health play a role in USMLE preparation?

Maintaining the mental and physical stamina required for USMLE preparation requires striking a balance between study time and personal well-being, which includes regular exercise, a good diet, and enough sleep.

Can technology help with preparing for the USMLE?

Indeed, technology can be an effective tool for preparing for the USMLE. Applications for time management, scheduling, and flashcards, as well as websites provide interactive materials that can improve your study effectiveness.

In the last weeks leading up to the USMLE exam, what should I concentrate on?

Reviewing important ideas, preparing with timed quizzes and practice tests, and making sure you are rested and psychologically ready for the test day should be your main priorities in the final weeks before the test.

Strategies to Help You Succeed on Step 1 of the USMLE

In medical school, you may always expect to study endlessly and take tests. One of the most challenging and demanding tests you will take throughout your time in medical school is the USMLE Step 1. In essence, how well you do on this test will determine whether you are successful or unsuccessful in the residency match procedure. Be assured that your USMLE Step 1 score is a major consideration for competitive residency programs as, in the majority of situations, it is the sole standardized and impartial assessment of your academic ability.

In essence, you need to perform well on this test. It indicates your ability to execute when it matters most, in addition to your discipline and capacity to absorb and integrate vast amounts of knowledge. I used all of the main study techniques, including First Aid, USMLE World, BRS, and Kaplan, when I took the Step 1 in 2009. Even though I felt well-prepared on test day, I was surprised by a couple parts of the exam. In the hopes that they would fully prepare you for the most significant test of your life, I have included some essential pearls below!

1. **lengthy question stems**

The length of the majority of the Step 1 questions was one of the most unexpected features. Even though I spent months studying extensively before the test, I was nonetheless rather taken aback. Even though I practiced a lot of example questions, the Step 1 questions were the longest I had ever encountered. To demonstrate the length of a typical exam question, the following sample question is provided:

A 45-year-old man with a thunderclap headache who has no noteworthy medical history arrives at the emergency room. When the patient complained of the "worst headache of his life" three hours before his presentation, he was in his typical state of health and consuming beer at home with a number of coworkers. He took acetaminophen and aspirin to treat his headache, but when the discomfort persisted, an ambulance took him to the hospital. His vital signs upon assessment are as follows: temperature: 37.5 °C; pulse: 75 bpm; blood pressure: 145/90 mm Hg; respiration rate: 10/minute; and pain level: 10/10. He is perceptive and aware of time, place, and people. Breath and heart sounds are typical. A neurologic examination is important for severe headaches, neck stiffness, and photophobia. Sensation and motor strength remain unaffected. In the case of renal tubular acidosis in the mother and diabetes and hypertension in the father, family history is important. For sporadic cocaine addiction, social history is important; the most recent instance occurred earlier today. The patient is a lawyer by profession. He does not take any prescriptions other than a daily multivitamin. There isn't any indication of bleeding on a non-contrast CT scan of the head. Both cocaine and marijuana are detected in urine.

CO_2: 21, BUN: 20, Creatinine: 1.1, Na: 141, K: 4.1, Cl: 120, and labs

CBC: WBC: 13K, Plt: 350K, Hb: 12.0, and Hct: 40

Coags: INR: 1.0, PT: 15, PTT: 35

To confirm a preliminary diagnosis of aneurysmal sub-arachnoid hemorrhage, a lumbar puncture is carried out.

WBC: 5, RBC: 30K, glucose: 100, protein: 120, OP: 30 cm H2O, and gram stain: no organisms. Color of CSF: xanthochromic.

A digital-subtraction angiography is performed on the patient once they are taken to the angio suite. He is sent right away to the operating room for microsurgical clip occlusion after being diagnosed with a ruptured posterior communicating aneurysm.

In the next 24 hours, which of the following is the biggest risk factor for aneurysm re-rupture?

The majority of exam questions are comparable to the sample above in terms of length and level of information. You are requesting a great deal of reading when you multiply this by 50 questions each section with several sections. It's very draining! As you can see, the question stems' body is crammed with irrelevant details that are meant to lead you astray. For the majority of diagnostic or clinical questions, you should anticipate receiving a complete set of vitals, lab results, and a thorough physical examination.

Reading what the test writers truly want you to answer at the bottom of the question stem is a crucial test-taking tactic. You can read the question stem again after you understand the direction of the inquiry. In this instance, it's likely that you can come up with an answer without even reading the stem.

Test Tips: Read the question itself by skimming to the bottom of the question stem. The question text is frequently useless and will merely take up time.

2. **Many Possible Answers**

The boards frequently offer a plethora of response options, making the process of elimination exceedingly challenging. Here is an example of the same question as before, along with a list of potential responses:

A 45-year-old man with a thunderclap headache who has no noteworthy medical history arrives at the emergency room. When the patient complained of the "worst headache of his life" three hours before his presentation, he was in his typical state of health and consuming beer at home with a number of coworkers. He took acetaminophen and aspirin to treat his headache, but when the discomfort persisted, an ambulance took him to the hospital. His vital signs upon assessment are as follows: temperature: 37.5 °C; pulse: 75 bpm; blood pressure: 145/90 mm Hg; respiration rate: 10/minute; and pain level: 10/10. He is perceptive and aware of time, place, and people. Breath and heart sounds are typical. A neurologic examination is important for severe headaches, neck stiffness, and photophobia. Sensation and motor strength remain unaffected. In the case of renal tubular acidosis in the mother and diabetes and hypertension in the father, family history is important. For sporadic cocaine addiction, social history is important; the most recent instance occurred earlier today. The patient is a lawyer by profession. He does not take any prescriptions other than a daily multivitamin. There isn't any indication of bleeding on a non-contrast CT scan of the head. Both cocaine and marijuana are detected in urine.

CO2: 21, BUN: 20, Creatinine: 1.1, Na: 141, K: 4.1, Cl: 120, and labs

CBC: WBC: 13K, Plt: 350K, Hb: 12.0, and Hct: 40

Coags: INR: 1.0, PT: 15, PTT: 35

To confirm a preliminary diagnosis of aneurysmal sub-arachnoid hemorrhage, a lumbar puncture is carried out.

WBC: 5, RBC: 30K, glucose: 100, protein: 120, OP: 30 cm H2O, and gram stain: no organisms. Color of CSF: xanthochromic.

A digital-subtraction angiography is performed on the patient once they are taken to the angio suite. He is sent right away to the operating room for microsurgical clip occlusion after being diagnosed with a ruptured posterior communicating aneurysm.

Which of the following is the greatest risk factor for aneurysm re-rupture in the next 24 hours?

A. History of recent cocaine abuse
B. Age < 50
C. Na > 140
D. CSF opening pressure > 20 cm H2O
E. WBC > 10K
F. Severe headache on presentation
H. Microsurgical clip occlusion of aneurysm
J. Unsecured cerebral aneurysm
G. RBC/WBC > 100
H. Microsurgical clip occlusion of aneurysm
I. Multivitamin Use
K. A and B
L. A and C
M. A, B, and D
O: All of the above
P: None of the above

There are many options, as you can see. The test-takers intentionally do this to interfere with your ability to identify the right response. You have a lengthy list of responses in addition to a lengthy question stem.

Test advice: The best course of action in this situation is to follow your "gut" instinct and do your best to exclude out response options. You must take a lot of practice exams and respond to a lot of sample questions if you want to feel at ease taking the boards.

3. **Biostatistics**

The inclusion of biostatistics on the boards has become increasingly important. This section of the test will be challenging unless you are quite familiar with concepts like positive predictive values, Kaplan-Meyer curves, hazard ratios, and number needed to treat (as it was for me). You will be required to quickly interpret obscure, intricate research that presents findings using unusual statistical techniques. I advise allocating a significant amount of your study time to practicing biostatistics problems and being familiar with the jargon and computations. The secret to performing well on Step 1 is this. The volume and complexity of the biostatistics questions that will be posed should not be understated.

Study biostatistics for test advice.

4. **Analyzing the outcomes of experiments**

A theoretical experiment will be used to illustrate a number of the pharmacology and physiology problems. Instead of asking you a straightforward question like "what enzyme is irreversibly inhibited by aspirin," the board examiners will ask you something more like this:

Three brand-new drugs (Compounds A, B, and C) are created by a scientist to treat coronary artery disease as a possible supplement to aspirin. In order to precisely monitor bleeding times, the scientist creates a platelet aggregation assay.

Medication	Bleeding Time
None	5 minutes
Aspirin	8 minutes
Compound A	8 minutes
Compound B	12 minutes
Compound C	15 minutes
Compound A+B	20 minutes
Compound A+C	8 minutes
Compound B+C	30 minutes

Based on the combination of medications above, Compound B exerts its mechanism of action most similarly to:

A. Aspirin 81 mg F. Apixaban K. A and C

B. Aspirin 325 mg G. Coumadin L. F and G

C. Clopidogrel H. Rivaroxaban M. A, B, and C

D. Prasugrel I. All of the above N. D and E

E. Bivalirudin J. None of the above O. G and H

Because these questions are challenging and test your ability to synthesize and grasp multiple topics at once, test examiners prefer to ask them. You must be familiar with the names, processes, and routes of almost all anti-platelet and anti-coagulant drugs in order to properly respond to these questions.

Test Advice: Ensure that you understand concepts like enzyme receptors and pharmaceutical modes of action. Keep in mind that these questions are frequently asked as part of an experiment rather than as a straightforward fact-recitation.

5. **There aren't many inquiries like "find the diagnosis."**

The Step 1 exam is fundamentally a basic scientific test. The majority of this test focuses on analyzing experiments, comprehending physiology and biochemistry, identifying histopathology slides, etc., while there will be a few clinical questions. You won't be asked to "choose the correct antibiotic(s) for ventilator-acquired pneumonia" or "what is the diagnosis?" during this exam. "type inquiries. These are the kinds of queries that are often saved for Steps two and three. Instead of researching the clinical signs and symptoms of bacterial endocarditis, concentrate on histology and mechanisms. Learn that cortisol is a steroid hormone that interacts to an intracellular receptor (as opposed to a cell membrane receptor) rather than analyzing how hypercortisolism results in the classic phenotypic symptoms of Cushing's disease.

Test Advice: Researching clinical questions, which are typically assessed on the Step 2, takes up most of your time. This is a common mistake. Practice questions should concentrate on genetics, biostatistics, experiments, routes, and processes. These are typically the subjects that undergo the most testing.

To sum up, Step 1 is challenging. Your success will mostly depend on the tried-and-true strategies of completing a large number of practice questions, studying effectively and early, and employing high-yield exam preparation books. Good luck, and work hard in your studies!

List of Abbreviations

Meaning of Abbreviations

Advanced Clinical Medicine (ACM)

American with Disabilities Act (ADA)

Bulletin of Information (BOI)

(CACMS) Committee on accreditation of Canada medical schools.

Candidate Identification Number (CIN)

Clinical Knowledge (CK)

Commission on Osteopathic College Accreditation (COCA)

Computers- based Case simulations (CCS)

(FLEX) Federation Licensing Examination

Federation of State Medical Boards (FSMB)

Foundations of Independent Practice (FIP)

Liaison Committee on Medical Education (LCME)

Multiple-choice questions, (MCQs)

United States Medical Licensing Examination (USMLE)

Laboratory Values

SERUM	Reference Range	SI Reference Intervals
General Chemistry:		
Electrolytes		
Sodium (Na+)	136–146 mEq/L	136–146 mmol/L
Potassium (K+)	3.5–5.0 mEq/L	3.5–5.0 mmol/L
Chloride (Cl−)	95–105 mEq/L	95–105 mmol/L
Bicarbonate (HCO$_3$)	22–28 mEq/L	22–28 mmol/L
Urea nitrogen	7–18 mg/dL	2.5–6.4 mmol/L
Creatinine	0.6–1.2 mg/dL	53–106 μmol/L
Glucose	Fasting: 70–100 mg/dL Random, non-fasting: <140 mg/dL	3.8–5.6 mmol/L <7.77 mmol/L
Calcium	8.4–10.2 mg/dL	2.1–2.6 mmol/L

Magnesium (Mg^{2+})	1.5–2.0 mg/dL	0.75–1.0 mmol/L
Phosphorus (inorganic)	3.0–4.5 mg/dL	1.0–1.5 mmol/L

Hepatic:

Alanine aminotransferase (ALT)	10–40 U/L	10–40 U/L
Aspartate aminotransferase (AST)	12–38 U/L	12–38 U/L
Alkaline phosphatase	25–100 U/L	25–100 U/L
Bilirubin, total // direct	0.1–1.0 mg/dL // 0.0–0.3 mg/dL	2–17 μmol/L // 0–5 μmol/L
Proteins, total	6.0–7.8 g/dL	60–78 g/L
Albumin	3.5–5.5 g/dL	35–55 g/L
Globulin	2.3–3.5 g/dL	23–35 g/L

Other, serum:

Amylase	25–125 U/L	25–125 U/L
Lipase	13–60 U/L	13–60 U/L
Creatinine clearance	Male: 97–137 mL/min Female: 88–128 mL/min	97–137 mL/min 88–128 mL/min
Creatine kinase	Male: 25–90 U/L Female: 10–70 U/L	25–90 U/L 10–70 U/L
Lactate dehydrogenase	45–200 U/L	45–200 U/L

Osmolality	275–295 mOsmol/kg H₂O	275–295 mOsmol/kg H₂O
Troponin I	≤0.04 ng/mL	≤0.04 µg/L
Uric Acid	3.0–8.2 mg/dL	0.18–0.48 mmol/L

Lipids:

Cholesterol

Total	Normal: <200 mg/dL High: >240 mg/dL	<5.2 mmol/L >6.2 mmol/L
HDL	40–60 mg/dL	1.0–1.6 mmol/L
LDL	<160 mg/dL	<4.2 mmol/L
Triglycerides	Normal: <150 mg/dL Borderline: 151–199 mg/dL	<1.70 mmol/L 1.71–2.25 mmol/L

Iron Studies:

Ferritin	Male: 20–250 ng/mL Female: 10–120 ng/mL	20–250 µg/L 10–120 µg/L
Iron	Male: 65–175 µg/dL Female: 50–170 µg/dL	11.6–31.3 µmol/L 9.0–30.4 µmol/L
Total iron-binding capacity	250–400 µg/dL	44.8–71.6 µmol/L
Transferrin	200–360 mg/dL	2.0–3.6 g/L

Endocrine:

Follicle-stimulating hormone	Male: 4–25 mIU/mL Female: premenopause 4–30 mIU/mL midcycle peak 10–90 mIU/mL postmenopause 40–250 mIU/mL	4–25 IU/L 4–30 IU/L 10–90 IU/L 40–250 IU/L
Luteinizing hormone	Male: 6–23 mIU/mL Female: follicular phase 5–30 mIU/mL midcycle 75–150 mIU/mL postmenopause 30–200 mIU/mL	6–23 IU/L 5–30 IU/L 75–150 IU/L 30–200 IU/L
Growth hormone - arginine stimulation	Fasting: <5 ng/mL Provocative stimuli: >7 ng/mL	<5 µg/L >7 µg/L
Prolactin (hPRL)	Male: <17 ng/mL Female: <25 ng/mL	<17 µg/L <25 µg/L
Cortisol	0800 h: 5–23 µg/dL 1600 h: 3–15 µg/dL 2000 h: <50% of 0800 h	138–635 nmol/L 82–413 nmol/L Fraction of 0800 h: <0.50

TSH	0.4–4.0 µU/mL	0.4–4.0 mIU/L
Triiodothyronine (T₃) (RIA)	100–200 ng/dL	1.5–3.1 nmol/L
Triiodothyronine (T₃) resin uptake	25%–35%	0.25–0.35
Thyroxine (T₄)	5–12 µg/dL	64–155 nmol/L
Free T₄	0.9–1.7 ng/dL	12.0–21.9 pmol/L
Thyroidal iodine (¹²³I) uptake	8%–30% of administered dose/24 h	0.08–0.30/24 h
Intact PTH	10–60 pg/mL	10–60 ng/L
17-Hydroxycorticosteroids	Male: 3.0–10.0 mg/24 h Female: 2.0–8.0 mg/24 h	8.2–27.6 µmol/24 h 5.5–22.0 µmol/24 h
17-Ketosteroids, total	Male: 8–20 mg/24 h Female: 6–15 mg/24 h	28–70 µmol/24 h 21–52 µmol/24 h

Immunoglobulins:

IgA	76–390 mg/dL	0.76–3.90 g/L
IgE	0–380 IU/mL	0–380 kIU/L
IgG	650–1500 mg/dL	6.5–15.0 g/L
IgM	50–300 mg/dL	0.5–3.0 g/L

GASES, ARTERIAL BLOOD (ROOM AIR)	Reference Range	SI Reference Intervals
PO_2	75–105 mm Hg	10.0–14.0 kPa
PCO_2	33–45 mm Hg	4.4–5.9 kPa
pH	7.35–7.45	[H$^+$] 36–44 nmol/L

CEREBROSPINAL FLUID	Reference Range	SI Reference Intervals
Cell count	0–5/mm^3	0–5 × 10^6/L
Chloride	118–132 mEq/L	118–132 mmol/L
Gamma globulin	3%–12% total proteins	0.03–0.12
Glucose	40–70 mg/dL	2.2–3.9 mmol/L
Pressure	70–180 mm H$_2$O	70–180 mm H$_2$O
Proteins, total	<40 mg/dL	<0.40 g/L

HEMATOLOGIC	Reference Range	SI Reference Intervals
Complete Blood Count:		
Hematocrit	Male: 41%–53% Female: 36%–46%	0.41–0.53 0.36–0.46
Hemoglobin, blood	Male: 13.5–17.5 g/dL Female: 12.0–16.0 g/dL	135–175 g/L 120–160 g/L
Mean corpuscular hemoglobin (MCH)	25–35 pg/cell	0.39–0.54 fmol/cell
Mean corpuscular hemoglobin conc. (MCHC)	31%–36% Hb/cell	4.8–5.6 mmol Hb/L
Mean corpuscular volume (MCV)	80–100 µm^3	80–100 fL
Volume		
Plasma	Male: 25–43 mL/kg Female: 28–45 mL/kg	0.025–0.043 L/kg 0.028–0.045 L/kg
Red cell	Male: 20–36 mL/kg Female: 19–31 mL/kg	0.020–0.036 L/kg 0.019–0.031 L/kg

Leukocyte count (WBC)	4500–11,000/mm³	4.5–11.0 × 10⁹/L
Neutrophils, segmented	54%–62%	0.54–0.62
Neutrophils, bands	3%–5%	0.03–0.05
Lymphocytes	25%–33%	0.25–0.33
Monocytes	3%–7%	0.03–0.07
Eosinophils	1%–3%	0.01–0.03
Basophils	0%–0.75%	0.00–0.0075
Platelet count	150,000–400,000/mm³	150–400 × 10⁹/L
Coagulation:		
Partial thromboplastin time (PTT/aPTT) (activated)	25–40 seconds	25–40 seconds
Prothrombin time (PT)	11–15 seconds	11–15 seconds
D-Dimer	≤250 ng/mL	≤1.4 nmol/L
Other, Hematologic:		
Reticulocyte count	0.5%–1.5%	0.005–0.015
Erythrocyte count (RBC)	Male: 4.3–5.9 million/mm³ Female: 3.5–5.5 million/mm³	4.3–5.9 × 10¹²/L 3.5–5.5 × 10¹²/L

Erythrocyte sedimentation rate (Westergren)	Male: 0-15 mm/h Female: 0-20 mm/h	0-15 mm/h 0-20 mm/h
CD4+ T-lymphocyte count	≥500/mm^3	≥0.5 × 10^9/L

Endocrine:

Hemoglobin A$_{1c}$	≤6%	≤42 mmol/mol

URINE	Reference Range	SI Reference Intervals
Calcium	100-300 mg/24 h	2.5-7.5 mmol/24 h
Osmolality	50-1200 mOsmol/kg H$_2$O	50-1200 mOsmol/kg H$_2$O
Oxalate	8-40 μg/mL	90-445 μmol/L
Proteins, total	<150 mg/24 h	<0.15 g/24 h

How to Create a Study Schedule for Step 1

To begin with, please be aware that there is no secret formula for performing well on the USMLE Step 1 exam. Some people can succeed fast with limited resources, while others require more help and take months. Although this test is crucial, it doesn't determine the type of doctor you will become. This test is merely an obstacle to be surmounted.

Recommended study duration for dedication:

6–8 weeks: To pass UWorld, you must complete at least 80 questions every day for seven weeks, totaling nearly 3500 questions. To get over your wrong questions a second time, I suggest attempting to complete a few more each day.

UWorld: The purpose of this question bank is to instruct you, not to assess your knowledge. It is your course manual. Don't worry about receiving a 40%; you will learn more the more mistakes you make.

First Aid: While answering Uworld questions, review First Aid.

Anki: The days of focusing on Anki all afternoon are long gone. Now, efficiency is crucial.

Pathoma: I regret not adhering to some of the more straightforward, high-yield elements there. First Aid and UWorld love to overwhelm you with information. Pathoma, STEP 1, and NBME are more likely to concentrate on prevalent diseases and high yield details.

Pixorize: This will assist you if you struggle with biochemistry. You don't want to overlook easy points because FTM has an exceptionally high yield.

Sketchy Medical: I pray to the "Sketchy Gods" even though I realize it's not for everyone. I still know every microorganism and antibiotic, even though it has been over three years since my USMLE Step 1 exam.

Time	Tasks	Comments
7am	breakfast/Anki	*Get your brain moving with some casual Anki. Hype music is a must (do not underestimate the power of some fun jams ♪).
8am	40 question UWORLD Block	Your Step exam is at 8am, so sit in your study space with your phone off and coffee brewed at 8am sharp. A little stress is good, get used to it. You'll be stressed on exam day.
9am	10 min break, fresh air	Get used to taking a break between every block, whether you think you need it or not. This will be required during test day.
9:10am	40 question UWORLD BLOCK	I like doing my second block right away, timed, not tutored. You MAY do blocks slower on tutor mode if you feel you learn better this way.
10:10am	10 min Coffee break	
		*NOTE: some days I recommend an extra 20-40 questions. Pushing yourself to 100 builds stamina and you simply get through the questions faster. I'd never do this the day before an NBME to keep my mind rested.
10:20am	Review 1st Block	It should take around 2-3 hours to properly review one block. Approximately 5 min per Question will take 3 hours. EVERY time you get a question wrong you should be finding/making Anki cards to add to your filter deck. THIS IS SO CRAZY IMPORTANT. I will post a video on filter decks later as well.
12pm	Lunch & ANKI	Anki contains incorrect questions or marked filter decks. Efficiency is key.
1pm	First Aid pages Biochem (3)/general principles(5)	Ideally done in a group, reading pages out loud. Ask each other questions, mention every UWorld question you've had on that topic. This should take around 6 min per page. Challenge each other.
2pm	Review 2nd UWorld block	Don't let fatigue set in. This second block is just as important as the first. Practice categorizing each question you get wrong into a knowledge problem or test taking problem.
4:30	30 minute exercise (cardio)	I know, how could you possibly make time for this? DO IT. Exercise builds neurons, gives you the only endorphins you're going to get during dedicated studying.
5:15	Dinner/Anki	
6pm	PATH/physio pages	Review topics/body systems you are weak in
7pm	Sketchy Medical /Pixorize	Priority goes to any micro or pharm Q you got wrong this day. If you get a question wrong on bisphosphonates, you must watch bisphosphonates.

Time	Tasks	Comments
8pm	Weaknesses	Worst subject cardio? Focus on this section with some review!
9pm	ANKI	Finish up wrongs/marked cards.
10pm	NETFLIX	Rest, relax. Have a couple Oreos <3.
11pm	SLEEP	LIGHTS OUT, phone in the other room. PRO-tip, listen to Golian audio to fall asleep. It's stronger than a benzo (can be found on Spotify).

To sum up,

First Aid for the USMLE is still among the most thorough and trustworthy materials available to medical students getting ready for the USMLE tests. It is a vital tool for understanding the key ideas covered in the tests because of its thorough material, succinct explanations, and well-structured format. Together with its useful advice and mnemonics, the book's emphasis on high-yield material gives pupils the best chance for success. Although it shouldn't be utilized as the only study aid, First Aid facilitates learning and increases retention when combined with other resources. It remains a pillar of the preparation process for students hoping to get high scores on the USMLE Step 1, Step 2 CK, and Step 3 exams.

Made in United States
North Haven, CT
13 June 2025

69794030R00128